AIP Diet for Beginners 2025

The Essential Guide to Healing Inflammation and Boosting Wellness with the Autoimmune Protocol

Sophia Harper

Disclaimer

The information provided in this book is for educational and informational purposes only and is not intended as a substitute for professional medical advice, diagnosis, or treatment. Always consult your physician, registered dietitian, or other qualified healthcare provider before making significant changes to your diet or lifestyle, especially if you have a medical condition, are pregnant, or are taking medications.

While every effort has been made to ensure the accuracy of the information presented, the author and publisher make no representations or warranties of any kind regarding the completeness, accuracy, or applicability of the content. Any reliance you place on the information provided in this book is strictly at your own risk.

The author and publisher disclaim any liability for any direct, indirect, or consequential loss or damage arising from the use of the material contained in this book.

Dedication

To all those seeking better health and a vibrant life, this book is for you. May it inspire positive changes, bring comfort, and help you on your journey toward wellness.

Table of Contents

Introduction

Welcome to *AIP diet for beginners 2025*. First, let me say this: you are not alone. Whether you're navigating the ups and downs of an autoimmune diagnosis, looking for ways to support someone you love, or simply seeking a healthier lifestyle, you've taken a brave step by picking up this book.

Living with an autoimmune condition can feel overwhelming at times. The unpredictable symptoms, the frustration of flare-ups, and the search for answers—it's a lot to manage. But here's the good news: there is hope. Some tools and strategies can help you regain control, and the Autoimmune Protocol (AIP) is one of them. This book is here to guide you, step by step, toward a path of healing and wellness.

Why This Book?

The purpose of this book is simple: to empower you with knowledge and actionable steps to manage your autoimmune condition effectively. The Autoimmune Protocol isn't just another "fad diet" or one-size-fits-all solution. It's a scientifically supported approach to reducing inflammation, healing the gut, and identifying triggers that may exacerbate autoimmune symptoms.

This journey isn't about deprivation or unrealistic goals—it's about giving your body the tools it needs to heal and thrive. Whether you're brand new to AIP or have tried bits and pieces before, this guide will break it all down for you in a way that feels approachable and achievable.

A Personal Note

I remember the first time I heard about the Autoimmune Protocol. A close friend had been struggling with debilitating symptoms from an autoimmune disease. She tried everything—medications, supplements, you name it—but nothing seemed to work. Then she discovered AIP. Within weeks of starting the protocol, she noticed a shift. Her energy improved, her flare-ups became less frequent, and she finally felt like she had control over her health again.

Her journey inspired me to dive deeper into AIP, not just for her sake but for others who might be searching for answers. Over time, I realized how transformative this approach could be—physically and emotionally. That's why I felt compelled to write this book: to share the tools, strategies, and hope that can come from embracing the Autoimmune Protocol.

What You'll Learn

This book is structured to give you everything you need to succeed with AIP, step by step. Here's what you can look forward to:

- **Understanding autoimmune conditions:** We'll start with the basics—what autoimmune diseases are, how they affect the body, and why diet and lifestyle changes can make such a difference.

- **The science behind AIP:** You'll learn how this protocol works, including its two key phases: elimination and reintroduction.

- **Practical steps to get started:** From stocking your pantry to planning your meals, I'll walk you through how to begin the protocol with confidence.

- **Lifestyle practices beyond food:** Healing isn't just about what you eat. We'll explore stress management, sleep, and movement as integral parts of your journey.

- **Recipes and meal plans:** You'll find a variety of delicious, easy-to-follow recipes to keep you inspired and nourished.

- **Tips for long-term success:** Finally, we'll discuss how to personalize AIP for your needs and maintain your progress over time.

A Journey Worth Taking

This book isn't about perfection. It's about progress. Healing is a deeply personal journey, and everyone's path will look a little different. Whether you're starting this protocol to manage a specific autoimmune condition or simply to improve your overall health, I hope that this guide will equip you with the tools, confidence, and support you need to succeed.

As you turn these pages, I invite you to approach this process with an open mind and a compassionate heart—both for yourself and your body. The fact that you're here, willing to learn and take action, is already a huge step forward. Together, let's explore the possibilities of what healing can look like for you.

Let's get started. Your path to empowered healing begins here.

Chapter 1

Understanding Autoimmune Diseases

Autoimmune diseases can feel like an unwelcome mystery, disrupting lives with little warning and often leaving those affected searching for answers. To take steps toward healing, it's essential to understand what these conditions are, why they happen, and how your daily choices—particularly regarding diet and lifestyle—play a role in managing them.

What Are Autoimmune Diseases?

An autoimmune disease occurs when the body's immune system, designed to protect you from harmful invaders like bacteria and viruses, mistakenly attacks its own healthy tissues. This "friendly fire" can lead to inflammation, damage, and dysfunction in various parts of the body.

For instance, think of your immune system as a security guard. Normally, it keeps intruders out while protecting what's inside. However, in autoimmune diseases, this guard becomes confused and starts attacking the very people it's supposed to protect.

Common Autoimmune Diseases and Symptoms

Autoimmune diseases are numerous, each affecting the body in different ways. Here are a few well-known examples:

- **Rheumatoid Arthritis (RA):** The immune system targets the joints, leading to pain, swelling, and stiffness, often in the hands and feet.

- **Hashimoto's Thyroiditis:** This condition affects the thyroid gland, often causing fatigue, weight gain, and sensitivity to cold.

- **Lupus (Systemic Lupus Erythematosus):** A complex disease that can impact the skin, joints, kidneys, and other organs, resulting in widespread symptoms like fatigue, joint pain, and rashes.

- **Type 1 Diabetes:** The immune system destroys insulin-producing cells in the pancreas, leading to problems regulating blood sugar.

- **Psoriasis:** This autoimmune condition causes skin cells to build up rapidly, forming scaly patches that can itch or hurt.

Although these diseases differ, they share one common feature: chronic inflammation. This persistent state of heightened immune activity plays a central role in their onset and progression.

The Role of Diet and Lifestyle in Autoimmune Health

Autoimmune diseases don't just appear overnight; they often develop from a combination of genetic predisposition and environmental factors. Among these, diet and lifestyle are some of the most powerful tools for managing symptoms and promoting overall health.

How Inflammation Impacts Autoimmune Conditions

Inflammation is a natural defense mechanism. If you've ever had a cut or infection, you've seen inflammation in action: redness, swelling, and heat are signs your body is fighting to heal.

But when inflammation becomes chronic, as is often the case in autoimmune diseases, it can harm the body instead of helping it. Persistent inflammation contributes to tissue damage, pain, and many of the symptoms associated with autoimmune conditions.

The Gut-Health Connection

The gut is often referred to as the "second brain," and for good reason. About 70% of your immune system resides in the gut, making its health a critical piece of the autoimmune puzzle.

The gut lining serves as a barrier, preventing harmful substances like undigested food particles and bacteria from entering the bloodstream. However, in individuals with autoimmune diseases, this barrier may become compromised— a condition known as "leaky gut."

When the gut barrier is weakened, toxins and other particles can pass through, triggering an immune response and fueling inflammation. This cycle of gut dysfunction and immune activation is why gut health is so vital in managing autoimmune conditions.

What Is the Autoimmune Protocol (AIP)?

The Autoimmune Protocol, or AIP, is a dietary and lifestyle framework specifically designed to help people with autoimmune diseases reduce inflammation, heal the gut, and identify foods that may be triggering their symptoms.

Definition and Purpose

AIP is not a one-size-fits-all diet but rather a structured process that focuses on nutrient-dense, anti-inflammatory foods while eliminating those that are known to irritate the immune system or gut. The protocol is divided into two key phases:

1. **Elimination Phase:** Foods that are common inflammatory triggers, such as gluten, dairy, grains, legumes, nuts, seeds, nightshade vegetables, and processed foods, are temporarily removed from the diet. This phase allows the body to reduce inflammation and begin healing.

2. **Reintroduction Phase:** Foods are gradually reintroduced one at a time to determine which ones are well-tolerated and which may need to be avoided in the long term.

The Science Behind AIP

The AIP framework is grounded in scientific principles. By focusing on whole, nutrient-rich foods and removing potential irritants, the protocol aims to:

- Lower inflammation throughout the body.

- Support gut healing by eliminating foods that compromise the gut lining.

- Provide essential nutrients to promote immune regulation and overall health.

The Gut-Health Connection

The AIP diet places significant emphasis on supporting gut health. Foods included in the protocol are chosen for their ability to repair the gut lining, reduce inflammation, and foster a healthy gut microbiome. Bone broth, fermented foods, and omega-3-rich fish are just a few examples of AIP-friendly choices that work to strengthen the gut and immune system simultaneously.

Why AIP Matters

For many, AIP is a lifeline—an opportunity to take control of their health in a world where autoimmune diseases often feel unpredictable and overwhelming. By addressing the root causes of inflammation and immune dysfunction, AIP offers more than just symptom management; it offers hope for long-term healing.

Now that we've explored what autoimmune diseases are and how AIP can help, the next step is diving into how you can begin implementing these strategies in your own life. In the following chapters, we'll cover practical steps to get started, from stocking your pantry to creating a personalized AIP plan that works for you. Let's continue on this journey to empowered health!

Chapter 2
What Is the Autoimmune Protocol (AIP)?

The Autoimmune Protocol (AIP) offers a practical, science-based approach to managing autoimmune conditions by addressing the root causes of inflammation and immune imbalance. It's not just a diet—it's a framework for healing that combines dietary changes, nutrient-rich foods, and lifestyle adjustments to help you regain control over your health.

The Foundations of AIP

The AIP diet is based on two core goals:

1. **Reducing Inflammation:** By removing common dietary triggers, AIP allows the body to calm the chronic inflammation that contributes to autoimmune symptoms.

2. **Identifying Food Sensitivities:** Through a structured process of elimination and reintroduction, AIP helps pinpoint which foods may be aggravating your condition.

The Two Phases of AIP

1. **Elimination Phase**

   The elimination phase is the heart of AIP. During this phase, certain foods that are known to trigger inflammation or irritate the immune system are temporarily removed from your diet. These include:

   o **Dairy** (e.g., milk, cheese, yogurt): Can irritate the gut lining and provoke immune responses.

   o **Grains** (e.g., wheat, oats, rice): Contain compounds like gluten that may trigger inflammation.

   o **Legumes** (e.g., beans, lentils, peanuts): Contain lectins and other compounds that can be challenging for some individuals.

   o **Nightshades** (e.g., tomatoes, potatoes, peppers): Contain alkaloids that may exacerbate inflammation.

   o **Processed and refined foods:** Often high in additives, sugars, and unhealthy fats, which can fuel inflammation.

This phase typically lasts 30-90 days, depending on individual needs. It provides a clean slate, giving your body the chance to reset and start healing.

2. **Reintroduction Phase**

Once symptoms have improved, foods are gradually reintroduced one at a time to determine how your body reacts. This phase requires patience and careful tracking.

For example, you might add back eggs by eating them for several days while monitoring for any changes in symptoms, such as digestive upset, joint pain, or skin reactions. If food causes symptoms, it may need to be avoided long-term, while others can be safely included in your diet.

The reintroduction phase empowers you to create a personalized eating plan that supports your health and minimizes autoimmune flare-ups.

How AIP Works

The effectiveness of AIP is rooted in its ability to calm the immune system and support overall healing.

The Science Behind AIP

When you remove inflammatory triggers from your diet, you reduce the burden on your immune system. This allows your body to repair damage, restore balance, and function more effectively.

The AIP diet also emphasizes gut health, which plays a central role in regulating the immune system. By healing the gut lining and fostering a diverse and balanced gut microbiome, AIP helps reduce the immune system's tendency to attack healthy tissues.

Benefits of AIP

Many people with autoimmune conditions report significant improvements while following AIP, including:

- Reduced joint pain and stiffness.
- Improved digestion and resolution of gut-related issues like bloating or diarrhea.
- Increased energy and reduced fatigue.
- Clearer skin and reduced rashes or flares.
- Enhanced mental clarity and mood stability.

While individual results vary, the protocol is designed to address the unique needs of each person, making it adaptable to various autoimmune conditions.

The Core Principles of AIP

AIP goes beyond simply eliminating harmful foods; it's also about adding nutrient-dense, healing foods that nourish the body.

Focus on Nutrient Density

Nutrient density refers to the concentration of vitamins, minerals, antioxidants, and other beneficial compounds in foods. The AIP diet prioritizes whole, unprocessed foods that supply your body with the tools it needs to repair and thrive.

Key nutrient-rich foods include:

- **Vegetables:** Especially leafy greens, cruciferous vegetables, and root vegetables.

- **Fruits:** Low-sugar options like berries, which are rich in antioxidants.

- **High-quality proteins:** Such as grass-fed meats, wild-caught fish, and organ meats.

- **Healthy fats:** Including coconut oil, olive oil, and avocados, which support cell repair and reduce inflammation.

- **Gut-healing foods:** Bone broth, fermented vegetables, and probiotics to strengthen the gut lining.

By focusing on nutrient-dense foods, AIP ensures your body has the raw materials needed for healing and long-term health.

A Path to Empowerment

The Autoimmune Protocol may seem restrictive at first, but its structured approach allows you to better understand your body and regain control over your health. AIP is not about deprivation—it's about discovering the foods and habits that support your well-being while identifying and avoiding what holds you back.

In the next chapter, we'll guide you through the practical steps of starting the AIP diet, from setting up your kitchen to planning your first AIP meals. Let's continue building this foundation of healing together.

Chapter 3

Core Principles of AIP

Transitioning to the Autoimmune Protocol (AIP) can feel like a big leap, but with a clear understanding of its principles, you'll be well-equipped to take charge of your health. This chapter focuses on the essential steps of the protocol: the elimination phase, the reintroduction phase, and embracing nutrient-dense foods. By understanding and applying these principles, you can create a sustainable approach to healing and wellness.

The Elimination Phase

The elimination phase is the foundation of AIP. During this phase, you temporarily remove foods that are known to trigger inflammation, disrupt gut health, or provoke autoimmune responses. While it might seem restrictive, this step is essential for giving your body a chance to heal and reset.

Foods to Avoid

Certain foods can irritate the immune system, even if they seem harmless. The following are excluded during the elimination phase:

- **Dairy:** Can disrupt gut health and contribute to inflammation.

- **Grains:** Contain gluten and other compounds that may irritate the digestive system.

- **Legumes:** Including beans, lentils, and peanuts, which contain lectins that can trigger immune reactions.

- **Nightshades:** Such as tomatoes, peppers, potatoes, and eggplants, which may aggravate inflammation for some people.

- **Processed and Refined Foods:** High in sugar, additives, and unhealthy fats, these foods promote inflammation and provide little nutritional value.

- **Nuts and Seeds:** Though healthy for some, these can be problematic for individuals with autoimmune conditions.

Why Avoid These Foods?

Each food category listed above contains compounds that can irritate the gut lining, disrupt hormone balance, or overstimulate the immune system. Removing these potential triggers allows your body to focus on healing without interference.

The Reintroduction Phase

After a period of elimination (usually 30-90 days), the reintroduction phase begins. This phase is about learning how your body reacts to specific foods so you can build a personalized diet that works for you.

Step-by-Step Guidance for Reintroduction

1. **Reintroduce One Food at a Time:** Choose a single food to reintroduce and consume it in small amounts for one day.

2. **Monitor Your Symptoms:** Pay close attention to how your body reacts over the next 72 hours. Watch for digestive issues, skin changes, joint pain, or fatigue.

3. **Wait Before Adding Another Food:** Allow a few days before testing another food to avoid confusing results.

Tips for Tracking Symptoms

- **Keep a Food Journal:** Note what you ate, the portion size, and any symptoms.

- **Be Patient:** Some reactions are subtle and may take time to identify.

This phase helps you understand which foods support your health and which ones may need to remain off-limits.

Nutrient-Dense Foods to Embrace

While the elimination phase focuses on avoiding triggers, the core of AIP emphasizes what you *can* eat. These foods are rich in the nutrients your body needs to heal and thrive.

Key Nutrients for Healing

- **Vitamins and Minerals:** Found abundantly in colorful vegetables and fruits.

- **Antioxidants:** Combat oxidative stress and reduce inflammation.

- **Healthy Fats:** Support cellular repair and hormone balance (e.g., avocado, coconut oil, olive oil).

- **Quality Proteins:** Aid tissue repair and immune function (e.g., grass-fed meats, wild-caught fish, organ meats).

AIP-Approved Foods

- **Vegetables:** Prioritize leafy greens, cruciferous vegetables, and root vegetables (excluding nightshades).

- **Fruits:** Low-sugar options like berries, which are packed with antioxidants.

- **Fermented Foods:** Sauerkraut, kimchi, and other fermented vegetables to support gut health.

- **Bone Broth:** A rich source of collagen and gut-healing compounds.

Eating a variety of these nutrient-dense foods ensures your body receives the essential building blocks for recovery.

Getting Started with AIP

Preparing Mentally and Physically

Starting AIP can feel overwhelming, but with preparation and the right mindset, it becomes manageable.

- **Set Realistic Goals:** Focus on progress, not perfection. Small steps can lead to significant changes.

- **Address Fears or Concerns:** It's normal to worry about giving up favorite foods or managing social situations. Remember, AIP is temporary and designed to help you feel better.

Stocking Your AIP Pantry

Having the right ingredients on hand makes AIP easier and more enjoyable.

- **AIP-Approved Staples:**
  - Fresh vegetables and fruits.
  - Quality proteins (grass-fed meats, wild-caught fish, organ meats).
  - Healthy fats (coconut oil, avocado oil, olive oil).
  - Herbs and spices (excluding nightshades like chili powder or paprika).
  - Fermented foods and bone broth.

- **Shopping Tips:**
  - Read labels carefully to avoid hidden additives or allergens.
  - Buy in bulk to save money on staples like coconut flour or cassava flour.

Meal Planning Basics

Planning meals ahead of time ensures you stay on track and reduces stress.

- **Balanced AIP Meals:** Combine a protein source, plenty of vegetables, and a healthy fat.

- **Sample Weekly Meal Plan:**
  - Breakfast: Sweet potato hash with sautéed greens and turkey sausage.
  - Lunch: Mixed green salad with grilled salmon and avocado.
  - Dinner: Roast chicken with roasted carrots and steamed broccoli.
  - Snacks: Fresh fruit or coconut yogurt.

Meal planning sets you up for success and makes AIP feel less restrictive.

A Framework for Healing

The core principles of AIP—eliminating triggers, reintroducing foods thoughtfully, and prioritizing nutrient-dense options—create a foundation for lasting health. With preparation and commitment, you'll be empowered to take control of your autoimmune journey and experience the benefits of reduced symptoms and improved well-being.

In the next chapter, we'll dive into practical lifestyle tips to complement your AIP journey, focusing on stress management, sleep, and exercise. Let's continue building a holistic path to healing together.

Chapter 4

AIP Lifestyle Beyond Food

While the Autoimmune Protocol (AIP) places a significant focus on diet, healing extends beyond what's on your plate. Your lifestyle plays an equally crucial role in managing autoimmune conditions. Stress, sleep, movement, and support systems can all influence your body's ability to heal and maintain balance. This chapter explores practical ways to integrate these components into your life to complement your AIP journey.

Stress Management

Chronic stress can have a significant impact on autoimmune conditions, exacerbating symptoms and slowing down healing. Learning how to manage stress effectively is a vital part of living well with autoimmune diseases.

Techniques to Reduce Stress

- **Meditation:** Dedicate a few minutes daily to mindfulness meditation. Apps or guided videos can help you get started.

- **Deep Breathing:** Simple breathing exercises, such as inhaling for four counts, holding for four, and exhaling for four, can quickly calm your nervous system.

- **Mindfulness Practices:** Stay present in the moment. Activities like journaling, drawing, or mindful walking can help you stay grounded.

- **Progressive Muscle Relaxation:** This involves tensing and then releasing each muscle group to ease physical and mental tension.

Practical Tips for Managing Stress

- **Set Boundaries:** Learn to say no to activities or commitments that overwhelm you.

- **Schedule Downtime:** Make relaxation a priority, even if it's just 10 minutes of quiet time each day.

- **Engage in Hobbies:** Spend time on activities that bring you joy and distraction from daily stressors.

Improving Sleep Quality

Sleep is one of the most powerful tools for healing. It's during sleep that your body repairs itself, balances hormones, and calms inflammation. Poor sleep, on the other hand, can worsen autoimmune symptoms.

Tips for Better Sleep Hygiene

- **Establish a Routine:** Go to bed and wake up at the same time every day, even on weekends.

- **Create a Restful Environment:** Keep your bedroom dark, cool, and quiet. Consider blackout curtains or a white noise machine if needed.

- **Limit Screen Time:** Avoid electronic devices at least an hour before bed. Blue light can disrupt your natural sleep rhythms.

- **Relax Before Bed:** Develop a calming pre-sleep routine, such as reading, taking a warm bath, or practicing gentle stretches.

- **Avoid Stimulants:** Reduce caffeine and heavy meals in the evening to promote better rest.

Why Sleep Is Essential for Healing

Sleep supports immune regulation, reduces inflammation, and helps your body recover from daily stressors. Even small improvements in sleep quality can lead to noticeable benefits in managing autoimmune symptoms.

Physical Activity

Exercise is important for overall health, but for those with autoimmune conditions, the type and intensity of physical activity matter. While too much strenuous exercise can increase inflammation, gentle and consistent movement can support healing and improve quality of life.

Types of Exercises Suitable for Autoimmune Conditions

- **Yoga:** Builds strength, improves flexibility, and promotes relaxation without overtaxing the body.

- **Walking:** A low-impact activity that boosts circulation, mood, and overall well-being.

- **Swimming:** Gentle on the joints and excellent for cardiovascular health.

- **Stretching or Tai Chi:** Enhances mobility and reduces stiffness while calming the mind.

Benefits of Gentle Movement

- Increases blood flow, delivering oxygen and nutrients to tissues.

- Supports lymphatic drainage to remove toxins.

- Enhances mental health by releasing endorphins and reducing stress.

Tips for Incorporating Movement

- Listen to Your Body: Some days, you may need to rest instead of exercise, and that's okay.

- Start Small: Begin with 10-minute sessions and gradually increase as your energy allows.

- Make It Fun: Choose activities you enjoy to stay consistent.

Building a Support System

Healing is not a solitary journey. Surrounding yourself with supportive people can make a world of difference in staying motivated and feeling understood.

How to Involve Family and Friends

- **Educate Them:** Share what AIP is and how it helps you manage your condition. Helping them understand your journey can foster empathy and support.

- **Ask for Help:** Whether it's meal prep, attending appointments, or emotional support, let them know how they can assist.

- **Set Boundaries:** Explain your needs kindly, such as avoiding certain foods at gatherings or respecting your need for rest.

Online Communities and Local Support Groups

- **Online Forums:** Join AIP or autoimmune-related groups on platforms like Facebook or Reddit. These communities can offer practical advice, recipe ideas, and moral support.

- **Local Groups:** Look for meetups or organizations in your area for people managing autoimmune conditions.

- **Professional Guidance:** Consider working with a coach, dietitian, or therapist familiar with AIP to keep you on track.

The Power of Connection

Knowing you're not alone in your journey can make challenges easier to face. Support systems provide encouragement, accountability, and a sense of belonging, all of which are vital for long-term success.

A Balanced Approach to Healing

Adopting AIP is not just about changing your diet—it's about creating a lifestyle that supports your well-being. By managing stress, prioritizing sleep, incorporating gentle movement, and building a strong support network, you're setting the stage for meaningful and lasting healing.

In the next chapter, we'll take a closer look at practical strategies for meal planning and preparation, ensuring that your transition to AIP is both smooth and enjoyable. Together, we'll continue this journey toward a healthier, more vibrant life.

Chapter 5

Troubleshooting Common Challenges

Starting and maintaining the Autoimmune Protocol (AIP) can be transformative, but it's not without its challenges. Life is full of moments that test our resolve—whether it's cravings, social situations, or unexpected flare-ups. This chapter offers practical strategies to help you navigate these hurdles while staying focused on your health goals.

Coping with Cravings and Setbacks

It's normal to experience cravings, especially when eliminating familiar foods. Setbacks are also a part of any long-term lifestyle change, and how you respond to them matters more than the setback itself.

Strategies to Stay on Track Without Feeling Deprived

1. **Focus on Abundance:** Shift your mindset from what you can't have to what you can enjoy. Explore the variety of AIP-friendly foods, flavors, and recipes available to you.

2. **Satisfy Cravings with Substitutes:**

   - Craving something sweet? Reach for fresh fruit like berries or try an AIP-friendly dessert.

   - Missing crunchy snacks? Try roasted veggie chips or kale crisps.

3. **Practice Mindful Eating:** Slow down and savor each bite. Mindful eating can help you feel more satisfied with smaller portions.

4. **Plan Ahead:** Anticipate situations that might lead to temptation, such as parties or stressful days. Keep AIP-approved snacks on hand to prevent impulsive choices.

5. **Practice Self-Compassion:** If you slip up, don't dwell on guilt or frustration. Acknowledge the moment, learn from it, and recommit to your goals.

Eating Out and Traveling on AIP

Social events, restaurant meals, and travel can feel intimidating when following AIP, but with preparation, you can navigate these situations with confidence.

Tips for Dining at Restaurants and Social Events

1. **Research the Menu:** Look up restaurant menus in advance to identify AIP-compliant options.

2. **Communicate Your Needs:** Politely explain your dietary requirements to servers or hosts. Most people are happy to accommodate when they understand your needs.

3. **Customize Orders:** Request simple dishes with grilled proteins, steamed vegetables, and healthy fats like olive oil. Ask for sauces or dressings on the side to avoid hidden ingredients.

4. **Eat Before You Go:** If you're unsure about available options, have a small AIP-friendly meal or snack beforehand to avoid arriving hungry.

5. **Bring a Dish:** For potlucks or gatherings, contribute an AIP-friendly dish that you and others can enjoy.

Packing AIP-Friendly Snacks for Travel

- **Non-Perishable Snacks:** Stock up on items like freeze-dried fruits, plantain chips, or compliant beef jerky.

- **Fresh Produce:** Pack easy-to-carry options like carrot sticks, apple slices, or mini cucumbers.

- **Homemade Options:** Prepare snack bars or energy bites using AIP-approved ingredients.

- **Stay Hydrated:** Bring a refillable water bottle and herbal teas to stay hydrated and curb hunger during travel.

Dealing with Flare-Ups

Despite your best efforts, flare-ups can happen. They're a reminder that autoimmune conditions can be unpredictable, but with the right strategies, you can minimize their impact and recover quickly.

Recognizing Triggers

1. **Keep a Journal:** Track your food, stress levels, sleep quality, and symptoms to identify potential patterns or triggers.

2. **Consider Hidden Factors:** Beyond food, triggers can include stress, lack of sleep, environmental factors, or even overexertion.

Managing Symptoms During a Flare-Up

1. **Rest and Recharge:** Give your body the time and space it needs to heal. Reduce physical and mental stressors.

2. **Return to Basics:** Stick to the elimination phase of AIP for a few days to calm inflammation and allow your body to reset.

3. **Hydrate:** Drink plenty of water to support detoxification and soothe your system. Herbal teas with anti-inflammatory properties, like ginger or chamomile, can also help.

4. **Seek Support:** Whether it's a friend, family member, or online AIP community, lean on others for encouragement and practical advice during tough times.

5. **Consult a Professional:** If flare-ups persist or worsen, consider seeking guidance from a healthcare provider or dietitian experienced in AIP.

A Journey, Not a Destination

Challenges are a natural part of any healing journey, but they don't define your success. Each step forward, no matter how small, brings you closer to your health goals. By developing practical coping strategies and learning from setbacks, you're equipping yourself to navigate the ups and downs of AIP with resilience.

Chapter 6

Breakfast Recipes

A nourishing breakfast sets the tone for your day, especially when following the Autoimmune Protocol (AIP). These recipes are designed to be nutrient-dense, flavorful, and easy to prepare, helping you kickstart your mornings with energy and confidence.

Sweet Potato Breakfast Hash

A hearty and nutritious breakfast hash made with sweet potatoes, onions, and herbs, perfect for a satisfying start to your day.

Estimated Meal Time

- **Prep and Cook:** 20 minutes

Ingredients

- 1 large sweet potato, diced
- ½ onion, chopped
- 1 tablespoon olive oil
- ½ teaspoon garlic powder (optional)
- Salt and pepper to taste

Cooking Method

1. In a skillet over medium heat, heat the olive oil.
2. Add diced sweet potato and cook for about 10-12 minutes until tender.
3. Add chopped onion, garlic powder, salt, and pepper. Stir well and cook for another 3–5 minutes.
4. Serve warm.

Nutritional Facts (per serving)

Calories: 180 | Protein: 3g | Carbs: 32g | Fat: 7g | Fiber: 5g

Portion Control

- 1 serving = 1 cup of hash.

Pro Tips

- For extra flavor, add fresh herbs like rosemary or thyme.

Apple Cinnamon Porridge

A warm, comforting porridge made with apples, cinnamon, and coconut milk for a cozy, grain-free breakfast.

Estimated Meal Time

- **Prep and Cook:** 10 minutes

Ingredients

- 1 apple, diced
- 1 cup coconut milk
- 1 tablespoon coconut flour
- 1 teaspoon cinnamon
- 1 tablespoon maple syrup (optional)

Cooking Method

1. In a saucepan, heat the coconut milk over medium heat.
2. Add diced apple, coconut flour, cinnamon, and maple syrup, stirring until the mixture thickens.
3. Simmer for 5-7 minutes, then serve warm.

Nutritional Facts (per serving)

Calories: 210 | Protein: 3g | Carbs: 30g | Fat: 12g | Fiber: 4g

Portion Control

- 1 serving = 1 cup of porridge.

Pro Tips

- Add chia seeds or flaxseeds for extra fiber.

Carrot and Parsnip Hash Browns

Crispy and golden hash browns made with carrots and parsnips, perfect for a savory breakfast.

Estimated Meal Time

- **Prep and Cook:** 15 minutes

Ingredients

- 1 large carrot, grated
- 1 large parsnip, grated
- 1 tablespoon olive oil
- Salt and pepper to taste

Cooking Method

1. Grate the carrot and parsnip.
2. In a skillet over medium heat, heat the olive oil.
3. Add the grated vegetables, pressing them into a flat layer in the skillet.
4. Cook for 3–5 minutes per side until golden and crispy.
5. Serve immediately.

Nutritional Facts (per serving)

Calories: 150 | Protein: 2g | Carbs: 25g | Fat: 7g | Fiber: 6g

Portion Control

- 1 serving = ½ cup of hash browns.

Pro Tips

- For added flavor, sprinkle with fresh parsley or chives.

AIP Banana Pancakes

Fluffy and naturally sweet banana pancakes, made without any grains or dairy, for a delightful breakfast treat.

Estimated Meal Time

- **Prep and Cook:** 10 minutes

Ingredients

- 1 ripe banana, mashed
- 2 eggs
- 1 tablespoon coconut flour
- 1 tablespoon coconut oil

Cooking Method

1. In a bowl, mash the banana until smooth.
2. Add eggs and coconut flour, stirring until combined.
3. Heat coconut oil in a skillet over medium heat.
4. Drop spoonfuls of batter into the skillet, cooking for 2–3 minutes per side.
5. Serve with fresh berries or coconut yogurt.

Nutritional Facts (per serving)

Calories: 210 | Protein: 6g | Carbs: 25g | Fat: 10g | Fiber: 4g

Portion Control

- 1 serving = 2 pancakes.

Pro Tips

- To keep pancakes warm, place them on a baking sheet in a low-temperature oven while you cook the rest.

Zucchini and Turkey Patties

Savory turkey patties mixed with zucchini, offering a protein-packed breakfast that's both light and filling.

Estimated Meal Time

- **Prep and Cook:** 15 minutes

Ingredients

- 1 cup zucchini, grated
- 1 pound ground turkey
- 1 tablespoon olive oil
- Salt and pepper to taste

Cooking Method

1. Grate zucchini and squeeze out excess moisture.
2. Mix zucchini with ground turkey, salt, and pepper.
3. Form mixture into patties.
4. In a skillet over medium heat, heat the olive oil.
5. Cook patties for 4–5 minutes per side, until golden and cooked through.
6. Serve warm.

Nutritional Facts (per serving)

Calories: 220 | Protein: 22g | Carbs: 5g | Fat: 14g | Fiber: 2g

Portion Control

- 1 serving = 2 patties.

Pro Tips

- Add fresh herbs like parsley or basil for extra flavor.

Coconut Yogurt with Berries

A creamy and refreshing breakfast made with dairy-free coconut yogurt and topped with antioxidant-rich berries.

Estimated Meal Time

- **Prep and Cook:** 5 minutes

Ingredients

- ½ cup coconut yogurt

- ½ cup mixed berries (such as blueberries, strawberries, or raspberries)

Cooking Method

1. Spoon coconut yogurt into a bowl.

2. Top with fresh berries.

3. Serve immediately.

Nutritional Facts (per serving)

Calories: 150 | Protein: 2g | Carbs: 18g | Fat: 10g | Fiber: 4g

Portion Control

- 1 serving = ½ cup of coconut yogurt with ½ cup of berries.

Pro Tips

- Add a drizzle of honey for natural sweetness.

Butternut Squash Breakfast Bowl

A warm, comforting breakfast bowl filled with roasted butternut squash, coconut milk, and a hint of cinnamon.

Estimated Meal Time

- **Prep and Cook:** 25 minutes

Ingredients

- 1 cup butternut squash, cubed
- ½ cup coconut milk
- 1 teaspoon cinnamon
- 1 tablespoon maple syrup (optional)

Cooking Method

1. Roast butternut squash at 400°F (200°C) for 20 minutes until tender.
2. In a bowl, combine roasted squash, coconut milk, cinnamon, and maple syrup.
3. Serve warm.

Nutritional Facts (per serving)

Calories: 220 | Protein: 2g | Carbs: 30g | Fat: 10g | Fiber: 6g

Portion Control

- 1 serving = 1 cup of the breakfast bowl.

Pro Tips

- Sprinkle with toasted coconut flakes for added crunch.

Plantain Waffles

These crispy, grain-free waffles are made with plantains for a naturally sweet and satisfying breakfast option.

Estimated Meal Time

- **Prep and Cook:** 20 minutes

Ingredients

- 2 ripe plantains, peeled
- 2 eggs
- 1 tablespoon coconut flour
- 1 teaspoon vanilla extract
- 1 tablespoon coconut oil (for greasing waffle iron)

Cooking Method

1. Blend the plantains in a food processor until smooth.
2. Add eggs, coconut flour, and vanilla extract. Blend again until fully combined.
3. Preheat the waffle iron and grease with coconut oil.
4. Pour the batter into the waffle iron and cook according to the manufacturer's instructions, about 4–5 minutes.
5. Serve with fresh fruit or coconut yogurt.

Nutritional Facts (per serving)

Calories: 250 | Protein: 5g | Carbs: 38g | Fat: 12g | Fiber: 6g

Portion Control

- 1 serving = 2 waffles.

Pro Tips

- For added crunch, sprinkle with chia or flax seeds.

Avocado and Bacon Bowl

A savory and satisfying breakfast bowl with creamy avocado, crispy bacon, and a touch of lemon.

Estimated Meal Time

- **Prep and Cook:** 10 minutes

Ingredients

- 1 ripe avocado, sliced

- 2 slices of bacon, cooked and crumbled

- 1 teaspoon lemon juice

- Salt and pepper to taste

Cooking Method

1. Cook bacon until crispy, then crumble it into small pieces.

2. Slice avocado and place it in a bowl.

3. Top with crumbled bacon, lemon juice, salt, and pepper.

4. Serve immediately.

Nutritional Facts (per serving)

Calories: 300 | Protein: 8g | Carbs: 12g | Fat: 26g | Fiber: 9g

Portion Control

- 1 serving = 1 avocado and 2 slices of bacon.

Pro Tips

- Add a sprinkle of nutritional yeast for a cheesy flavor without dairy.

Cassava Flour Crepes

Thin, delicate crepes made with cassava flour, perfect for filling with AIP-friendly ingredients like berries or coconut cream.

Estimated Meal Time

- **Prep and Cook:** 15 minutes

Ingredients

- ½ cup cassava flour

- 2 eggs

- ½ cup coconut milk

- 1 tablespoon coconut oil

- A pinch of salt

Cooking Method

1. Whisk together cassava flour, eggs, coconut milk, and salt until smooth.

2. Heat a non-stick skillet over medium heat and lightly grease with coconut oil.

3. Pour ¼ cup of batter into the skillet, swirling to coat the bottom of the pan.

4. Cook for 1-2 minutes per side until golden.

5. Serve with fresh berries or coconut cream.

Nutritional Facts (per serving)

Calories: 180 | Protein: 6g | Carbs: 18g | Fat: 10g | Fiber: 3g

Portion Control

- 1 serving = 2 crepes.

Pro Tips

- Fill with your favorite AIP-friendly fruit for a sweet treat.

Roasted Veggie Breakfast Bake

A nourishing, savory bake filled with roasted vegetables and topped with eggs for a protein-packed breakfast.

Estimated Meal Time

- **Prep and Cook:** 30 minutes

Ingredients

- 1 cup bell peppers, chopped
- 1 cup zucchini, chopped
- 1 cup cherry tomatoes, halved
- 1 tablespoon olive oil
- 4 eggs
- Salt and pepper to taste

Cooking Method

1. Preheat the oven to 375°F (190°C).
2. Toss the chopped vegetables in olive oil, salt, and pepper, then roast in the oven for 20 minutes.
3. Crack eggs on top of the roasted vegetables and bake for another 10 minutes, or until eggs are set.
4. Serve warm.

Nutritional Facts (per serving)

Calories: 220 | Protein: 12g | Carbs: 20g | Fat: 14g | Fiber: 6g

Portion Control

- 1 serving = 1 egg and 1 cup of roasted vegetables.

Pro Tips

- Add fresh herbs like parsley or cilantro for a burst of freshness.

Beef and Kale Breakfast Skillet

A savory skillet of seasoned beef and kale makes for a hearty, nutrient-dense breakfast.

Estimated Meal Time

- **Prep and Cook:** 15 minutes

Ingredients

- 1/2 pound ground beef
- 2 cups kale, chopped
- 1 tablespoon olive oil
- 1 teaspoon garlic powder
- Salt and pepper to taste

Cooking Method

1. In a skillet over medium heat, heat the olive oil.
2. Add ground beef and cook until browned, breaking it up as it cooks.
3. Add kale, garlic powder, salt, and pepper. Cook for another 3–4 minutes until the kale wilts.
4. Serve immediately.

Nutritional Facts (per serving)

Calories: 350 | Protein: 30g | Carbs: 8g | Fat: 24g | Fiber: 3g

Portion Control

- 1 serving = 1/2 cup beef and 1 cup kale.

Pro Tips

- Use grass-fed beef for a richer flavor and additional health benefits.

Cabbage and Sausage Stir-Fry

This stir-fry combines cabbage and sausage for a deliciously savory, filling breakfast.

Estimated Meal Time

- **Prep and Cook:** 20 minutes

Ingredients

- 2 cups cabbage, shredded
- 2 sausages (AIP-friendly), sliced
- 1 tablespoon coconut oil
- Salt and pepper to taste

Cooking Method

1. Heat coconut oil in a skillet over medium heat.
2. Add sliced sausage and cook until browned.
3. Add shredded cabbage and cook for 5-7 minutes, stirring occasionally until tender.
4. Season with salt and pepper, then serve warm.

Nutritional Facts (per serving)

Calories: 280 | Protein: 18g | Carbs: 12g | Fat: 20g | Fiber: 6g

Portion Control

- 1 serving = 1 cup of stir-fry.

Pro Tips

- For added flavor, try using sage or thyme when cooking the sausage.

Tigernut Granola with Coconut Milk

A crunchy and nutty granola made from tiger nuts, perfect for an AIP-compliant breakfast with coconut milk.

Estimated Meal Time

- **Prep and Cook:** 20 minutes

Ingredients

- 1 cup tiger nuts
- ½ cup shredded coconut (unsweetened)
- 2 tablespoons coconut oil
- 1 teaspoon cinnamon
- 1 tablespoon honey (optional)
- 1 cup coconut milk

Cooking Method

1. Preheat the oven to 350°F (175°C).
2. Toss tiger nuts and shredded coconut in melted coconut oil, cinnamon, and honey (if using).
3. Spread the mixture on a baking sheet and bake for 15 minutes, stirring halfway through.
4. Serve the granola with coconut milk.

Nutritional Facts (per serving)

Calories: 180 | Protein: 3g | Carbs: 22g | Fat: 12g | Fiber: 6g

Portion Control

- 1 serving = ½ cup granola with ½ cup coconut milk.

Pro Tips

- For a sweeter touch, drizzle with additional honey or maple syrup before serving.

Pumpkin Breakfast Porridge

A warming, autumn-inspired porridge made with pumpkin, perfect for starting your day on a cozy note.

Estimated Meal Time

- **Prep and Cook:** 15 minutes

Ingredients

- ½ cup pumpkin puree
- 1 cup coconut milk
- 2 tablespoons chia seeds
- 1 teaspoon cinnamon
- 1 teaspoon vanilla extract
- A pinch of salt

Cooking Method

1. In a small saucepan, combine pumpkin puree, coconut milk, chia seeds, cinnamon, vanilla, and salt.
2. Bring to a simmer and cook for 5-7 minutes, stirring occasionally.
3. Once thickened, remove from heat and serve warm.

Nutritional Facts (per serving)

Calories: 220 | Protein: 5g | Carbs: 18g | Fat: 15g | Fiber: 6g

Portion Control

- 1 serving = 1 cup of porridge.

Pro Tips

- Top with extra chia seeds or a sprinkle of cinnamon for added texture and flavor.

Cauliflower Rice Breakfast Bowl

A savory breakfast bowl made with cauliflower rice, avocado, and bacon—
perfect for a low-carb, AIP-compliant meal.

Estimated Meal Time

- **Prep and Cook:** 15 minutes

Ingredients

- 2 cups cauliflower rice

- 1 avocado, sliced

- 2 slices bacon, cooked and crumbled

- Salt and pepper to taste

- 1 tablespoon olive oil

Cooking Method

1. In a skillet over medium heat, heat the olive oil.

2. Add cauliflower rice and cook for 5-7 minutes, stirring occasionally.

3. Season with salt and pepper.

4. Top with sliced avocado and crumbled bacon. Serve immediately.

Nutritional Facts (per serving)

Calories: 250 | Protein: 10g | Carbs: 16g | Fat: 20g | Fiber: 7g

Portion Control

- 1 serving = 1 cup cauliflower rice with 1/2 avocado and 2 slices of bacon.

Pro Tips

- For extra flavor, add a squeeze of lemon juice over the avocado.

Bone Broth with Greens

A nutrient-dense breakfast that provides healing and soothing properties, perfect for boosting your immune system.

Estimated Meal Time

- **Prep and Cook:** 10 minutes

Ingredients

- 2 cups bone broth (AIP-friendly)

- 1 cup spinach or kale, chopped

- 1 clove garlic, minced

- Salt and pepper to taste

Cooking Method

1. In a small pot, bring bone broth to a simmer.

2. Add the garlic and chopped greens and cook for 3–4 minutes until the greens wilt.

3. Season with salt and pepper. Serve hot.

Nutritional Facts (per serving)

Calories: 120 | Protein: 10g | Carbs: 4g | Fat: 8g | Fiber: 2g

Portion Control

- 1 serving = 2 cups of bone broth with greens.

Pro Tips

- Add a splash of lemon juice or apple cider vinegar for extra flavor and digestive support.

Salmon and Avocado Wraps (in lettuce)

A light and healthy breakfast with omega-3-rich salmon and creamy avocado, wrapped in lettuce for a refreshing bite.

Estimated Meal Time

- **Prep and Cook:** 10 minutes

Ingredients

- 4 oz cooked salmon (or canned salmon)
- 1 avocado, sliced
- 4 large lettuce leaves (romaine or butter lettuce works best)
- Salt and pepper to taste
- Lemon wedges for serving

Cooking Method

1. Warm the salmon if necessary, then break it into chunks.
2. Place the lettuce leaves on a plate, then layer with salmon and avocado slices.
3. Season with salt, pepper, and a squeeze of lemon juice.
4. Serve immediately as wraps or open-faced.

Nutritional Facts (per serving)

Calories: 280 | Protein: 22g | Carbs: 10g | Fat: 20g | Fiber: 7g

Portion Control

- 1 serving = 2 lettuce wraps.

Pro Tips

- For added flavor, drizzle with olive oil or add fresh herbs like cilantro.

AIP-Friendly Smoothie Bowl

A colorful smoothie bowl packed with antioxidants and healthy fats, perfect for starting your day with a nutrient boost.

Estimated Meal Time

- **Prep and Cook:** 10 minutes

Ingredients

- 1 cup frozen berries (blueberries, raspberries, etc.)
- ½ cup coconut milk (or water for lighter consistency)
- 1 tablespoon chia seeds
- ½ banana
- 2 tablespoons shredded coconut (unsweetened)

Cooking Method

1. Blend the frozen berries, coconut milk, chia seeds, and banana until smooth.
2. Pour the smoothie into a bowl and top with shredded coconut and extra berries.
3. Serve immediately.

Nutritional Facts (per serving)

Calories: 220 | Protein: 3g | Carbs: 28g | Fat: 14g | Fiber: 8g

Portion Control

- 1 serving = 1 smoothie bowl.

Pro Tips

- For added crunch, top with sliced almonds or sunflower seeds.

Herb-Seasoned Chicken Patties

These flavorful chicken patties are a great breakfast option that can be paired with a salad or avocado.

Estimated Meal Time

- **Prep and Cook:** 20 minutes

Ingredients

- 1 lb ground chicken
- 1 teaspoon garlic powder
- 1 teaspoon onion powder
- 1 teaspoon dried thyme
- 1 tablespoon olive oil
- Salt and pepper to taste

Cooking Method

1. In a bowl, combine ground chicken, garlic powder, onion powder, thyme, salt, and pepper.
2. Create little patties out of the mixture.
3. In a skillet over medium heat, heat the olive oil.
4. Cook the patties for 5-6 minutes on each side until golden and cooked through.
5. Serve with a side of greens or on their own.

Nutritional Facts (per serving)

Calories: 250 | Protein: 22g | Carbs: 1g | Fat: 18g | Fiber: 1g

Portion Control

- 1 serving = 2 patties.

Pro Tips

- Make a batch and store leftovers for a quick breakfast throughout the week.

These recipes offer a variety of AIP-friendly breakfast options, perfect for providing balanced nutrition while supporting your autoimmune healing journey. Enjoy!

Lunch Recipes

Lunch is an opportunity to fuel your body with nutrient-rich foods that will keep you energized and satisfied throughout the day. These AIP-friendly lunch recipes are designed to be simple, delicious, and nourishing, helping you stick to your autoimmune protocol while enjoying a variety of flavors.

Grilled Chicken with Roasted Vegetables

A healthy and satisfying meal featuring grilled chicken paired with roasted seasonal vegetables.

Estimated Meal Time:

- **30 minutes** (prep and cook)

Ingredients:

- 2 boneless, skinless chicken breasts

- 1 tbsp olive oil

- 1 tsp sea salt

- ½ tsp black pepper (optional)

- 1 red bell pepper, cut into chunks

- 1 zucchini, sliced

- 1 cup broccoli florets

- 1 tbsp dried thyme

Cooking Method:

1. Preheat the grill to medium-high heat.

2. Rub chicken breasts with olive oil, sea salt, pepper, and thyme.

3. Grill chicken for 6–7 minutes per side, or until internal temperature reaches 165°F.

4. While grilling, toss vegetables with olive oil, salt, and pepper, and roast in the oven at 400°F for 20 minutes or until tender.

5. Serve the grilled chicken with roasted vegetables.

Nutritional Facts (per serving):

Calories: 310 | Protein: 35g | Carbs: 15g | Fat: 14g | Fiber: 5g

Substitution Variations:

- Replace chicken with turkey or fish.

- Use other vegetables like asparagus, mushrooms, or sweet potatoes.

- Add a drizzle of AIP-friendly pesto for extra flavor.

Portion Control:

- One serving includes one chicken breast and 1 ½ cups of vegetables.

Pro Tips:

- Marinate the chicken in olive oil, lemon, and herbs for 30 minutes for enhanced flavor.

- For a smoky flavor, try grilling the vegetables alongside the chicken.

AIP Beef Stir-Fry with Bell Peppers

A quick and flavorful stir-fry featuring tender beef and colorful bell peppers, making it perfect for an AIP-friendly lunch.

Estimated Meal Time:

- **20 minutes** (prep and cook)

Ingredients:

- 1 lb grass-fed beef, sliced thin
- 2 tbsp olive oil
- 2 bell peppers, sliced
- 1 onion, sliced
- 2 cloves garlic, minced
- 1 tbsp coconut aminos
- 1 tsp dried oregano
- 1 tsp sea salt

Cooking Method:

1. Heat olive oil in a large skillet over medium-high heat.
2. Add sliced beef and cook for 4–5 minutes until browned.
3. Remove beef from skillet and set aside.
4. In the same skillet, add bell peppers, onion, and garlic, and cook for 3–4 minutes until softened.
5. Return beef to the skillet, add coconut aminos, oregano, and salt, and stir well.
6. Cook for an additional 2 minutes. Serve hot.

Nutritional Facts (per serving):

Calories: 320 | Protein: 28g | Carbs: 12g | Fat: 18g | Fiber: 4g

Substitution Variations:

- Replace beef with chicken or pork.
- Add other veggies like zucchini, mushrooms, or spinach.
- Use tamari sauce instead of coconut aminos for a different flavor.

Portion Control:

- One serving includes 4 oz of beef and 1 cup of vegetables.

Pro Tips:

- Use grass-fed beef for a leaner cut.
- Serve with a side of cauliflower rice for a complete meal.

Salmon and Avocado Salad

A fresh, nutrient-packed salad featuring grilled salmon and creamy avocado, perfect for a light lunch.

Estimated Meal Time:

- **15 minutes** (prep and cook)

Ingredients:

- 2 salmon fillets
- 1 tbsp olive oil
- 1 tsp sea salt
- ½ tsp black pepper (optional)
- 1 avocado, diced
- 2 cups mixed greens
- 1 tbsp olive oil (for salad dressing)
- 1 tbsp lemon juice

Cooking Method:

1. Preheat grill or skillet to medium-high heat.
2. Rub salmon fillets with olive oil, sea salt, and pepper.
3. Grill salmon for 4–5 minutes per side until the internal temperature reaches 145°F.
4. In a bowl, toss mixed greens with diced avocado, olive oil, and lemon juice.
5. Flake the salmon and top the salad with it. Serve immediately.

Nutritional Facts (per serving):

Calories: 350 | Protein: 30g | Carbs: 8g | Fat: 25g | Fiber: 6g

Substitution Variations:

- Replace salmon with tuna or grilled chicken.
- Add other salad toppings like cucumbers or radishes.
- Use lime juice instead of lemon for a different citrus flavor.

Portion Control:

- One serving includes 1 salmon fillet and 2 cups of salad.

Pro Tips:

- For extra flavor, drizzle AIP-friendly dressing, like olive oil and balsamic vinegar, on top.
- Make the salad ahead of time and add the salmon just before serving to keep it fresh.

Chicken and Sweet Potato Soup

A hearty, comforting soup filled with tender chicken and sweet potatoes, making it an ideal AIP-friendly meal.

Estimated Meal Time:

- **40 minutes** (prep and cook)

Ingredients:

- 2 boneless, skinless chicken breasts, cubed
- 2 medium sweet potatoes, peeled and diced
- 1 tbsp olive oil
- 1 onion, diced
- 2 cloves garlic, minced
- 4 cups chicken broth (AIP-friendly)
- 1 tsp sea salt
- 1 tsp ground cinnamon
- 1 tsp dried thyme

Cooking Method:

1. In a large pot, heat olive oil over medium heat. Add onion and garlic, and cook for 2–3 minutes.
2. Add cubed chicken and cook for 5–6 minutes until browned.
3. Stir in sweet potatoes, chicken broth, sea salt, cinnamon, and thyme.
4. Bring to a boil, then reduce heat and simmer for 20–25 minutes, or until sweet potatoes are tender.
5. Serve hot.

Nutritional Facts (per serving):

Calories: 280 | Protein: 25g | Carbs: 30g | Fat: 10g | Fiber: 6g

Substitution Variations:

- Use turkey instead of chicken.
- Add other vegetables like carrots or parsnips.
- Use bone broth for extra richness.

Portion Control:

- One serving includes 1 ½ cups of soup.

Pro Tips:

- Blend half of the soup for a creamier texture.

- Serve with a side of AIP-friendly bread for a more filling meal.

AIP Turkey Lettuce Wraps

These delicious wraps feature seasoned turkey in crisp lettuce, perfect for a light and refreshing meal.

Estimated Meal Time:

- **20 minutes** (prep and cook)

Ingredients:

- 1 lb ground turkey
- 1 tbsp olive oil
- 1 onion, finely chopped
- 1 clove garlic, minced
- 1 tbsp coconut aminos
- 1 tsp ground cumin
- 1 tsp paprika
- Salt and pepper to taste
- 8 large lettuce leaves (such as butter lettuce or romaine)

Cooking Method:

1. In a skillet, heat the olive oil over medium heat. Add onion and garlic, and sauté for 2–3 minutes.

2. Add ground turkey and cook until browned, breaking it up with a spoon.

3. Stir in coconut aminos, cumin, paprika, salt, and pepper. Cook for another 3–4 minutes.

4. Spoon turkey mixture onto lettuce leaves, wrap, and serve.

Nutritional Facts (per serving):

Calories: 250 | Protein: 30g | Carbs: 5g | Fat: 14g | Fiber: 2g

Substitution Variations:

- Use ground chicken or beef instead of turkey.
- Add chopped avocado or cucumber to the wraps for extra freshness.
- Use coconut wraps instead of lettuce for a different texture.

Portion Control:

- One serving includes 2 wraps.

Pro Tips:

- For added flavor, top with AIP-friendly salsa or guacamole.
- Serve with a side of roasted sweet potato for a more filling meal.

Zucchini Noodles with Ground Beef and Tomato Sauce

A satisfying, low-carb dish featuring zucchini noodles topped with a rich ground beef and tomato sauce.

Estimated Meal Time:

- **25 minutes** (prep and cook)

Ingredients:

- 2 medium zucchinis, spiralized
- 1 lb ground beef
- 1 tbsp olive oil
- 1 can (14.5 oz) crushed tomatoes
- 1 tsp dried oregano
- 1 tsp garlic powder
- Salt and pepper to taste
- Fresh basil for garnish (optional)

Cooking Method:

1. Heat olive oil in a skillet over medium-high heat. Add ground beef and cook, breaking it up as it browns.

2. Stir in crushed tomatoes, oregano, garlic powder, salt, and pepper. Simmer for 10 minutes.

3. While the sauce simmers, sauté zucchini noodles in a separate pan with olive oil for 2–3 minutes until tender.

4. Serve the zucchini noodles topped with the beef and tomato sauce, garnished with fresh basil.

Nutritional Facts (per serving):

Calories: 300 | Protein: 27g | Carbs: 12g | Fat: 18g | Fiber: 4g

Substitution Variations:

- Use turkey or pork instead of beef.
- Replace zucchini noodles with spaghetti squash or cauliflower rice.
- Add spinach or mushrooms to the tomato sauce for extra veggies.

Portion Control:

- One serving includes 1 cup of zucchini noodles and 1 ½ cups of sauce.

Pro Tips:

- For a creamier texture, add a tablespoon of AIP-friendly coconut milk to the sauce.

- To make zucchini noodles less watery, lightly salt them and let them sit for 10 minutes before cooking.

Cauliflower Rice and Shrimp Stir-Fry

This flavorful stir-fry pairs shrimp with cauliflower rice, offering a light and healthy AIP-friendly meal.

Estimated Meal Time:

- **20 minutes** (prep and cook)

Ingredients:

- 1 lb shrimp, peeled and deveined
- 1 tbsp olive oil
- 1 cup cauliflower rice (store-bought or homemade)
- 1 bell pepper, sliced
- 1 carrot, julienned
- 2 cloves garlic, minced
- 1 tbsp coconut aminos
- 1 tsp ground ginger
- Salt and pepper to taste

Cooking Method:

1. Heat olive oil in a large skillet over medium heat. Cook the shrimp for two to three minutes on each side, or until they are opaque and pink. Remove from skillet and set aside.

2. In the same skillet, add cauliflower rice, bell pepper, and carrot. Sauté for 3–4 minutes until vegetables soften.

3. Stir in garlic, coconut aminos, ginger, salt, and pepper, and cook for 1–2 minutes.

4. Return shrimp to the skillet and stir everything together. Serve hot.

Nutritional Facts (per serving):

Calories: 280 | Protein: 30g | Carbs: 14g | Fat: 12g | Fiber: 5g

Substitution Variations:

- Replace shrimp with chicken, turkey, or beef.
- Add other vegetables like zucchini or mushrooms to the stir-fry.
- Use tamari instead of coconut aminos for a different flavor.

Portion Control:

- One serving includes 4 oz of shrimp and 1 ½ cups of cauliflower rice stir-fry.

Pro Tips:

- For extra flavor, add a sprinkle of fresh cilantro before serving.

- Serve with a side of roasted sweet potatoes for a more filling meal.

AIP Eggplant and Beef Stew

A hearty stew filled with tender beef and eggplant, simmered in a rich broth and perfect for an AIP-friendly meal.

Estimated Meal Time:

- **45 minutes** (prep and cook)

Ingredients:

- 1 lb stew beef, cubed
- 1 tbsp olive oil
- 1 onion, diced
- 2 cloves garlic, minced
- 2 eggplants, diced
- 4 cups beef broth (AIP-friendly)
- 1 tsp dried rosemary
- 1 tsp sea salt
- 1 tsp ground black pepper (optional)

Cooking Method:

1. Heat olive oil in a large pot over medium-high heat. Add stew beef and brown on all sides.
2. Add onion and garlic, and sauté for 2–3 minutes until softened.
3. Stir in diced eggplant, beef broth, rosemary, sea salt, and pepper.
4. Bring to a boil, then reduce heat and simmer for 30 minutes or until beef is tender.
5. Serve hot.

Nutritional Facts (per serving):

Calories: 320 | Protein: 28g | Carbs: 18g | Fat: 14g | Fiber: 7g

Substitution Variations:

- Use lamb or pork instead of beef.
- Add other vegetables like carrots or celery to the stew.
- Use bone broth for extra richness.

Portion Control:

- One serving includes 1 ½ cups of stew.

Pro Tips:

- For a thicker stew, mash some of the eggplant before serving.

- Serve with AIP-friendly crackers or bread on the side.

Grilled Pork Chops with Apple Slaw

A savory and tangy dish featuring perfectly grilled pork chops paired with a refreshing apple slaw.

Estimated Meal Time:

- **30 minutes** (prep and cook)

Ingredients:

- 4 boneless pork chops
- 1 tbsp olive oil
- 1 tsp dried thyme
- Salt and pepper to taste
- 2 apples, julienned
- 1 cup shredded cabbage
- ½ cup shredded carrots
- 2 tbsp olive oil
- 1 tbsp apple cider vinegar
- 1 tsp honey (optional)

Cooking Method:

1. Preheat the grill to medium-high heat.
2. Rub pork chops with olive oil, thyme, salt, and pepper. Grill for 4–5 minutes per side, until cooked through.
3. While pork chops are grilling, mix apples, cabbage, and carrots in a large bowl.
4. In a separate bowl, whisk together olive oil, apple cider vinegar, and honey. Pour over the slaw and toss to coat.
5. Serve pork chops with a generous serving of apple slaw.

Nutritional Facts (per serving):

Calories: 350 | Protein: 30g | Carbs: 22g | Fat: 20g | Fiber: 5g

Substitution Variations:

- Use chicken breasts or thighs instead of pork chops.
- Add raisins or cranberries to the apple slaw for a sweet touch.

- Use cabbage slaw mix instead of making it from scratch.

Portion Control:

- One serving includes 1 pork chop and 1 cup of apple slaw.

Pro Tips:

- For a smokier flavor, try grilling the pork chops with wood chips.

- Prepare the slaw ahead of time and store it in the fridge to allow the flavors to meld.

Coconut Curry Chicken with Spinach

A rich and creamy coconut curry paired with tender chicken and fresh spinach for a delicious and comforting meal.

Estimated Meal Time:

- **35 minutes** (prep and cook)

Ingredients:

- 1 lb chicken breast, cubed
- 1 tbsp coconut oil
- 1 onion, chopped
- 2 cloves garlic, minced
- 1 can (14 oz) coconut milk (AIP-friendly)
- 1 tbsp curry powder
- 1 tsp ground turmeric
- 1 tsp ground ginger
- 4 cups fresh spinach
- Salt and pepper to taste

Cooking Method:

1. Heat coconut oil in a large skillet over medium heat. Add chicken and cook until browned. Remove chicken and set aside.

2. In the same skillet, sauté onion and garlic until softened, about 3–4 minutes.

3. Stir in curry powder, turmeric, and ginger, and cook for 1 minute.

4. Add coconut milk and bring to a simmer. Return chicken to the skillet and cook for 10–15 minutes, until chicken is cooked through.

5. Stir in spinach and cook until wilted, about 2–3 minutes. Season with salt and pepper, and serve hot.

Nutritional Facts (per serving):

Calories: 350 | Protein: 30g | Carbs: 12g | Fat: 22g | Fiber: 4g

Substitution Variations:

- Use bone-in chicken thighs for more flavor.

- Add cauliflower or sweet potatoes for extra vegetables.

- Replace spinach with kale or Swiss chard.

Portion Control:

- One serving includes 4 oz of chicken and 1 cup of curry sauce.

Pro Tips:

- For a milder curry, reduce the amount of curry powder and ginger.

- Serve over cauliflower rice or AIP-friendly rice for a complete meal.

AIP Chicken and Veggie Skewers

Grilled chicken and colorful vegetables on skewers, make a fun and delicious AIP-friendly meal.

Estimated Meal Time:

- **25 minutes** (prep and cook)

Ingredients:

- 1 lb chicken breast, cut into 1-inch cubes
- 1 bell pepper, chopped
- 1 zucchini, chopped
- 1 red onion, chopped
- 1 tbsp olive oil
- 1 tsp dried oregano
- 1 tsp garlic powder
- Salt and pepper to taste

Cooking Method:

1. Preheat the grill to medium-high heat.
2. Thread chicken and vegetables onto skewers, alternating pieces.
3. Drizzle with olive oil and sprinkle with oregano, garlic powder, salt, and pepper.
4. Grill for 6–8 minutes per side, or until the chicken is cooked through and vegetables are tender.
5. Serve hot.

Nutritional Facts (per serving):

Calories: 280 | Protein: 35g | Carbs: 15g | Fat: 12g | Fiber: 4g

Substitution Variations:

- Use beef or lamb instead of chicken.
- Add mushrooms, cherry tomatoes, or asparagus to the skewers for added flavor.
- Serve with a side of AIP-friendly dipping sauce or guacamole.

Portion Control:

- One serving includes 3 skewers.

Pro Tips:

- Soak wooden skewers in water for 30 minutes before grilling to prevent burning.

- Marinate the chicken in olive oil and herbs for 30 minutes for extra flavor.

Roasted Salmon with Asparagus

A simple yet delicious roasted salmon dish paired with perfectly roasted asparagus for a healthy and flavorful meal.

Estimated Meal Time:

- **25 minutes** (prep and cook)

Ingredients:

- 4 salmon fillets
- 1 tbsp olive oil
- 1 bunch asparagus, trimmed
- 1 tsp garlic powder
- 1 tsp dried thyme
- Salt and pepper to taste

Cooking Method:

1. Preheat oven to 400°F (200°C).
2. Place salmon fillets and asparagus on a baking sheet. Sprinkle with salt, pepper, thyme, and garlic powder after drizzling with olive oil.
3. Roast for 15–20 minutes, until salmon is cooked through and asparagus is tender.
4. Serve immediately.

Nutritional Facts (per serving):

Calories: 350 | Protein: 30g | Carbs: 8g | Fat: 22g | Fiber: 4g

Substitution Variations:

- Use trout, cod, or any other firm white fish instead of salmon.
- Add lemon slices on top of the salmon before roasting for extra flavor.
- Serve with a side of cauliflower rice or roasted sweet potatoes.

Portion Control:

- One serving includes 1 fillet of salmon and 1 cup of asparagus.

Pro Tips:

- For a crispier texture, broil the salmon for the last 2–3 minutes of cooking.
- For extra flavor, drizzle with AIP-friendly pesto or lemon dressing before serving.

AIP Chicken Salad with Avocado

A fresh and creamy chicken salad with ripe avocado and crisp vegetables, perfect for a light and satisfying lunch.

Estimated Meal Time:

- **15 minutes** (prep)

Ingredients:

- 2 cups cooked chicken, shredded
- 1 avocado, diced
- 1 cucumber, chopped
- 1 cup mixed greens
- 1 tbsp olive oil
- 1 tbsp apple cider vinegar
- Salt and pepper to taste

Cooking Method:

1. In a large bowl, combine shredded chicken, avocado, cucumber, and mixed greens.
2. Drizzle with olive oil and apple cider vinegar, and toss to combine.
3. Season with salt and pepper to taste, and serve immediately.

Nutritional Facts (per serving):

Calories: 320 | Protein: 30g | Carbs: 10g | Fat: 22g | Fiber: 6g

Substitution Variations:

- Add sliced bell peppers or tomatoes for more vegetables.
- Use chicken thighs instead of chicken breasts for more flavor.
- Add a hard-boiled egg or bacon for extra protein.

Portion Control:

- One serving includes 1 cup of chicken salad.

Pro Tips:

- Make the salad ahead of time and refrigerate for up to 2 days.
- For extra creaminess, add a dollop of AIP-friendly mayo or coconut yogurt.

Sweet Potato and Ground Turkey Bowl

A hearty and flavorful bowl with roasted sweet potatoes and seasoned ground turkey, perfect for meal prep or a quick dinner.

Estimated Meal Time:

- **30 minutes** (prep and cook)

Ingredients:

- 2 medium sweet potatoes, peeled and cubed
- 1 lb ground turkey
- 1 tbsp olive oil
- 1 tsp cumin
- 1 tsp paprika
- ½ tsp garlic powder
- Salt and pepper to taste
- 2 cups spinach, chopped

Cooking Method:

1. Preheat oven to 400°F (200°C).
2. Toss sweet potato cubes with olive oil, salt, and pepper. Roast for 20–25 minutes, until tender.
3. While the sweet potatoes are roasting, heat a pan over medium heat and cook ground turkey until browned, breaking it apart as it cooks.
4. Add cumin, paprika, garlic powder, salt, and pepper to the turkey, and cook for 1–2 more minutes.
5. Stir in spinach and cook until wilted, about 2–3 minutes.
6. Serve the turkey mixture over roasted sweet potatoes.

Nutritional Facts (per serving):

Calories: 400 | Protein: 35g | Carbs: 30g | Fat: 20g | Fiber: 8g

Substitution Variations:

- Use ground chicken, beef, or lamb instead of turkey.
- Add roasted bell peppers or zucchini for extra veggies.
- Replace spinach with kale or arugula.

Portion Control:

- One serving includes 1 cup of sweet potatoes and 1 cup of turkey mixture.

Pro Tips:

- For extra flavor, top with avocado or a drizzle of olive oil.

- Make a large batch for meal prep and store in the fridge for up to 4 days.

AIP-Friendly Chicken Soup with Greens

A warm, nourishing chicken soup made with AIP-compliant ingredients and packed with greens for a comforting meal.

Estimated Meal Time:

- **40 minutes** (prep and cook)

Ingredients:

- 1 lb chicken breast, cubed
- 4 cups bone broth or chicken broth (AIP-friendly)
- 2 carrots, sliced
- 2 celery stalks, chopped
- 1 onion, chopped
- 2 cups spinach or kale
- 1 tbsp olive oil
- 1 tsp dried thyme
- Salt and pepper to taste

Cooking Method:

1. In a large pot, heat olive oil over medium heat. Add chicken and cook until browned, about 5–6 minutes.
2. Add carrots, celery, and onion, and cook for an additional 3–4 minutes.
3. Pour in bone broth and bring to a boil. Reduce heat and simmer for 20–25 minutes, until vegetables are tender.
4. Stir in spinach or kale, and cook for 3–5 minutes until wilted.
5. Season with thyme, salt, and pepper, and serve hot.

Nutritional Facts (per serving):

Calories: 280 | Protein: 30g | Carbs: 12g | Fat: 12g | Fiber: 4g

Substitution Variations:

- Use any AIP-compliant vegetables, such as zucchini, parsnips, or turnips.
- Add coconut milk for a creamier texture.
- Substitute chicken with turkey or beef for variety.

Portion Control:

- One serving includes 1 ½ cups of soup.

Pro Tips:

- Make a double batch and freeze extra servings for later.
- For a spicier kick, add fresh ginger or a pinch of turmeric.

Sautéed Shrimp and Squash

A light and flavorful dish with shrimp sautéed with summer squash, making a quick and satisfying AIP-friendly meal.

Estimated Meal Time:

- **20 minutes** (prep and cook)

Ingredients:

- 1 lb shrimp, peeled and deveined
- 2 medium squashes, sliced
- 2 tbsp olive oil
- 1 tsp garlic powder
- 1 tsp dried basil
- Salt and pepper to taste

Cooking Method:

1. Heat olive oil in a large skillet over medium-high heat.
2. Add shrimp and cook for 2–3 minutes per side until pink and cooked through. Remove shrimp and set aside.
3. In the same skillet, add squash slices and sauté for 4–5 minutes, until tender.
4. Add shrimp back to the pan with garlic powder, basil, salt, and pepper. Cook for another 1–2 minutes to combine flavors.
5. Serve hot.

Nutritional Facts (per serving):

Calories: 250 | Protein: 30g | Carbs: 10g | Fat: 14g | Fiber: 4g

Substitution Variations:

- Use zucchini or yellow squash instead of summer squash.
- Add diced bell peppers for extra flavor.
- Serve over cauliflower rice or mashed sweet potatoes for a heartier meal.

Portion Control:

- One serving includes 4 oz of shrimp and 1 cup of squash.

Pro Tips:

- For extra flavor, drizzle with lemon juice or AIP-friendly pesto before serving.
- Add fresh herbs like parsley or cilantro for a burst of color and taste.

Lemon Herb Chicken with Broccoli

A simple yet flavorful dish with grilled chicken seasoned with lemon and herbs, paired with steamed broccoli for a nutritious and satisfying meal.

Estimated Meal Time:

- **25 minutes** (prep and cook)

Ingredients:

- 2 chicken breasts
- 1 tbsp olive oil
- Juice of 1 lemon
- 1 tsp dried thyme
- 1 tsp dried rosemary
- Salt and pepper to taste
- 2 cups broccoli florets, steamed

Cooking Method:

1. Preheat the grill or a grill pan over medium heat.
2. In a small bowl, combine olive oil, lemon juice, thyme, rosemary, salt, and pepper.
3. Rub the seasoning mixture onto the chicken breasts and grill for 6–7 minutes on each side until fully cooked.
4. While the chicken cooks, steam the broccoli until tender.
5. Serve the grilled chicken alongside the steamed broccoli.

Nutritional Facts (per serving):

Calories: 320 | Protein: 35g | Carbs: 10g | Fat: 15g | Fiber: 5g

Substitution Variations:

- Use chicken thighs instead of breasts for a juicier option.
- Replace broccoli with asparagus, green beans, or sautéed spinach.
- Add a side of sweet potatoes for extra carbs.

Portion Control:

- One serving includes 1 chicken breast and 1 cup of steamed broccoli.

Pro Tips:

- Marinate the chicken for 30 minutes to intensify the flavor.
- Drizzle with extra lemon juice just before serving for added freshness.

AIP Stuffed Bell Peppers

A colorful and healthy dish with bell peppers stuffed with a savory combination of ground meat and vegetables, perfect for a balanced AIP-friendly meal.

Estimated Meal Time:

- **35 minutes** (prep and cook)

Ingredients:

- 4 bell peppers, tops cut off and seeds removed
- 1 lb ground beef or turkey
- 1 medium zucchini, chopped
- 1 medium onion, chopped
- 1 tbsp olive oil
- 1 tsp garlic powder
- 1 tsp dried oregano
- Salt and pepper to taste

Cooking Method:

1. Preheat the oven to 375°F (190°C).
2. In a skillet, heat olive oil over medium heat and sauté onion and zucchini until soft, about 5 minutes.
3. Add ground meat, garlic powder, oregano, salt, and pepper, cooking until browned and fully cooked.
4. Place the bell peppers in a baking dish after stuffing them with the meat mixture.
5. Cover with foil and bake for 20 minutes, then uncover and bake for an additional 5 minutes until the peppers are tender.
6. Serve hot.

Nutritional Facts (per serving):

Calories: 300 | Protein: 30g | Carbs: 12g | Fat: 18g | Fiber: 6g

Substitution Variations:

- Use ground chicken or lamb instead of beef.
- Add diced tomatoes or mushrooms to the stuffing mix for extra flavor.

- Top with a sprinkle of nutritional yeast for a cheesy flavor.

Portion Control:

- One serving includes 1 stuffed bell pepper.

Pro Tips:

- Make extra stuffing and store it in the fridge for easy meals later.

- For a spicier kick, add diced jalapeños or chili flakes to the stuffing.

Baked Cod with Roasted Carrots

A light and flavorful meal with baked cod paired with roasted carrots, making a nutritious and easy-to-prepare dinner.

Estimated Meal Time:

- **30 minutes** (prep and cook)

Ingredients:

- 4 cod fillets
- 4 large carrots, peeled and sliced
- 2 tbsp olive oil
- 1 tsp garlic powder
- 1 tsp paprika
- Salt and pepper to taste

Cooking Method:

1. Preheat the oven to 400°F (200°C).
2. Place the carrots on a baking sheet, drizzle with olive oil, and season with salt, pepper, garlic powder, and paprika. Roast for 20–25 minutes until tender.
3. Meanwhile, place cod fillets on a separate baking sheet, drizzle with olive oil, and season with salt, pepper, and paprika. Bake for 12–15 minutes until the fish is flaky.
4. Serve the baked cod with roasted carrots.

Nutritional Facts (per serving):

Calories: 280 | Protein: 25g | Carbs: 20g | Fat: 14g | Fiber: 6g

Substitution Variations:

- Use any white fish such as tilapia or haddock in place of cod.
- Roast other vegetables like sweet potatoes, parsnips, or Brussels sprouts alongside the carrots.
- Add a squeeze of lemon juice on top of the cod for extra flavor.

Portion Control:

- One serving includes 1 cod fillet and 1 cup of roasted carrots.

Pro Tips:

- For a crispy texture, broil the cod for the last 2 minutes of cooking.
- Season with fresh herbs like parsley or dill before serving for added flavor.

AIP Tuna Salad with Cucumber and Olives

A fresh and tangy tuna salad with crunchy cucumber and olives, perfect for a light lunch or as a snack.

Estimated Meal Time:

- **10 minutes** (prep)

Ingredients:

- 1 can tuna in water, drained
- 1 cucumber, diced
- 1/4 cup black olives, pitted and chopped
- 2 tbsp olive oil
- 1 tbsp apple cider vinegar
- Salt and pepper to taste

Cooking Method:

1. In a bowl, combine tuna, cucumber, and olives.
2. Drizzle with olive oil and apple cider vinegar, and Mix to blend.
3. Season with salt and pepper, and serve immediately.

Nutritional Facts (per serving):

Calories: 250 | Protein: 30g | Carbs: 6g | Fat: 14g | Fiber: 2g

Substitution Variations:

- Use avocado instead of olive oil for a creamier texture.
- Add chopped celery or green onions for extra crunch.
- Replace olives with capers for a tangy twist.

Portion Control:

- One serving includes 1/2 can of tuna salad.

Pro Tips:

- This salad can be prepared in advance and stored in the fridge for up to 2 days.
- Serve with AIP-friendly crackers or lettuce leaves for a satisfying meal.

These recipes offer a variety of AIP-friendly lunch options, perfect for providing balanced nutrition while supporting your autoimmune healing journey. Enjoy!

Dinner Recipes

These dinner recipes are carefully designed to offer AIP-friendly options that are both nourishing and satisfying. Each dish is rich in flavors and made with wholesome ingredients that support your autoimmune healing process. Enjoy these meals that are not only delicious but also beneficial for your health.

Herb-Crusted Chicken with Roasted Brussels Sprouts

A satisfying dish featuring succulent herb-crusted chicken paired with crispy roasted Brussels sprouts, this recipe is a perfect AIP-friendly dinner.

Estimated Meal Time:

- 30 minutes (prep and cook)

Ingredients:

- 4 boneless, skinless chicken breasts
- 2 tbsp olive oil
- 1 tbsp dried rosemary
- 1 tbsp dried thyme
- 1 tsp garlic powder
- Salt and pepper to taste
- 2 cups Brussels sprouts, trimmed and halved

Cooking Method:

1. Preheat oven to 400°F (200°C).

2. Rub chicken breasts with olive oil and season with rosemary, thyme, garlic powder, salt, and pepper.

3. Arrange chicken breasts on a baking sheet and place halved Brussels sprouts around them.

4. Roast in the oven for 20–25 minutes until the chicken reaches an internal temperature of 165°F (74°C) and the Brussels sprouts are crispy.

5. Serve immediately.

Nutritional Facts (per serving): Calories: 350 | Protein: 35g | Carbs: 20g | Fat: 18g | Fiber: 8g

Substitution Variations:

- Use chicken thighs for a juicier alternative
- Swap Brussels sprouts for other roasted vegetables like cauliflower or carrots.

Portion Control:

- A 4 oz chicken breast is typically one serving. Adjust the amount of Brussels sprouts based on personal preference—about 1 cup per serving.

Pro Tips:

- To enhance flavor, add a squeeze of fresh lemon juice on top of the chicken before serving.
- If you like your Brussels sprouts extra crispy, increase the roasting time by a few minutes.

Grilled Salmon with Garlic Mashed Cauliflower

A flavorful salmon fillet served with creamy garlic mashed cauliflower—a healthy, low-carb alternative to mashed potatoes.

Estimated Meal Time:

- 30 minutes (prep and cook)

Ingredients:

- 2 salmon fillets
- 2 tbsp olive oil
- 2 cloves garlic, minced
- 1 medium cauliflower, cut into florets
- 1/4 cup coconut milk
- Salt and pepper to taste

Cooking Method:

1. Preheat the grill to medium-high heat.
2. Brush the salmon fillets with olive oil and season with salt and pepper. Grill the salmon for 4–6 minutes per side, or until the internal temperature reaches 145°F (63°C).
3. While the salmon is cooking, steam the cauliflower florets for 8–10 minutes until tender.
4. Mash the steamed cauliflower with garlic and coconut milk until smooth. Season with salt and pepper.
5. Serve the grilled salmon with a side of garlic-mashed cauliflower.

Nutritional Facts (per serving): Calories: 420 | Protein: 30g | Carbs: 15g | Fat: 30g | Fiber: 7g

Substitution Variations:

- Try using other fish such as tilapia or cod for a lighter option.
- Substitute mashed cauliflower with mashed sweet potatoes for a different flavor.

Portion Control:

- One 4 oz salmon fillet is a standard serving. For cauliflower, about 1 cup of mashed cauliflower per serving works well.

Pro Tips:

- Add a sprinkle of fresh herbs such as dill or parsley to the mashed cauliflower for extra flavor.
- If you prefer creamier mashed cauliflower, add more coconut milk until the desired consistency is reached.

AIP Beef and Sweet Potato Stew

This hearty and comforting stew is packed with tender beef, sweet potatoes, and vegetables, making it a filling and nutritious AIP-friendly dish.

Estimated Meal Time:

- 1 hour (prep and cook)

Ingredients:

- 1 lb beef stew meat
- 2 tbsp olive oil
- 1 onion, chopped
- 2 cloves garlic, minced
- 2 large sweet potatoes, peeled and cubed
- 4 cups AIP-compliant broth
- 1 tsp dried thyme
- Salt and pepper to taste

Cooking Method:

1. Heat olive oil in a large pot over medium heat. Brown the beef stew meat in batches, then set aside.
2. In the same pot, sauté onion and garlic until softened, about 5 minutes.
3. Add the sweet potatoes, broth, thyme, and browned beef. Bring to a boil.
4. Reduce the heat to low and simmer for 45 minutes to 1 hour, until the beef is tender and the sweet potatoes are cooked through.
5. Season with salt and pepper to taste. Serve warm.

Nutritional Facts (per serving): Calories: 350 | Protein: 30g | Carbs: 30g | Fat: 15g | Fiber: 6g

Substitution Variations:

- Use lamb or chicken for a different protein option.
- Add other root vegetables like carrots or parsnips for extra flavor and texture.

Portion Control:

- A typical serving size is 1.5 cups of stew, or about 4 oz of beef with 1 cup of sweet potatoes. Adjust based on personal preferences.

Pro Tips:

- To add depth of flavor, add a splash of AIP-compliant vinegar or lemon juice just before serving.
- This stew can be made in advance and stored in the fridge for up to 3 days, or frozen for longer storage.

Baked Chicken Thighs with Roasted Vegetables

Tender and juicy baked chicken thighs paired with a colorful mix of roasted vegetables make for a quick and easy dinner.

Estimated Meal Time:

- 40 minutes (prep and cook)

Ingredients:

- 4 bone-in, skin-on chicken thighs
- 2 tbsp olive oil
- 1 tsp paprika
- 1/2 tsp garlic powder
- Salt and pepper to taste
- 2 cups mixed vegetables (carrots, zucchini, bell peppers, etc.)

Cooking Method:

1. Preheat oven to 375°F (190°C).
2. Rub the chicken thighs with olive oil, paprika, garlic powder, salt, and pepper.
3. Arrange chicken thighs on a baking sheet and surround them with mixed vegetables.
4. Roast for 35 to 40 minutes, or until the veggies are soft and the chicken reaches an internal temperature of 165°F (74°C).
5. Serve immediately.

Nutritional Facts (per serving): Calories: 400 | Protein: 30g | Carbs: 18g | Fat: 25g | Fiber: 6g

Substitution Variations:

- Substitute chicken breasts for a leaner protein.
- Use any variety of vegetables, such as broccoli or cauliflower, for a different flavor.

Portion Control:

- A single chicken thigh (about 4 oz) is typically one serving. Adjust the vegetable portion based on preference—about 1 cup of roasted vegetables per serving is recommended.

Pro Tips:

- For crispier chicken skin, broil the chicken for the last 3–5 minutes of cooking.
- Serve with a side of leafy greens for added nutrients.

Zucchini Noodles with Shrimp and Avocado

A light, refreshing dish with zucchini noodles paired with succulent shrimp and creamy avocado—this recipe is both satisfying and AIP-friendly.

Estimated Meal Time:

- 20 minutes (prep and cook)

Ingredients:

- 4 medium zucchinis, spiralized into noodles
- 1 lb shrimp, peeled and deveined
- 1 avocado, diced
- 2 tbsp olive oil
- 2 cloves garlic, minced
- 1 tsp lemon zest
- Salt and pepper to taste
- Fresh parsley for garnish (optional)

Cooking Method:

1. Heat olive oil in a large skillet over medium heat. Add garlic and sauté until fragrant, about 1 minute.
2. Add shrimp and cook for 3–4 minutes per side, until pink and cooked through. Remove shrimp from the skillet and set aside.
3. In the same skillet, sauté zucchini noodles for 2–3 minutes until tender.
4. Toss the zucchini noodles with shrimp, avocado, lemon zest, salt, and pepper.
5. Garnish with fresh parsley and serve immediately.

Nutritional Facts (per serving): Calories: 320 | Protein: 25g | Carbs: 15g | Fat: 22g | Fiber: 7g

Substitution Variations:

- Use chicken or scallops as a protein alternative to shrimp.
- Add cherry tomatoes or spinach for more vegetables.

Portion Control:

- A typical serving consists of 1 ½ cups of zucchini noodles and 4 oz of shrimp. Adjust portions based on appetite.

Pro Tips:

- For extra flavor, drizzle some lemon juice or olive oil over the dish before serving.
- If you prefer a thicker sauce, add a tablespoon of coconut milk to the skillet after cooking the shrimp.

AIP Braised Lamb with Root Vegetables

This tender braised lamb dish is cooked low and slow with a medley of root vegetables, making for a flavorful and comforting meal.

Estimated Meal Time:

- 2 hours (prep and cook)

Ingredients:

- 1 lb lamb shoulder, cut into chunks
- 2 tbsp olive oil
- 1 onion, chopped
- 2 cloves garlic, minced
- 4 large carrots, peeled and chopped
- 2 parsnips, peeled and chopped
- 3 cups AIP-compliant broth
- 1 tsp dried rosemary
- 1 tsp thyme
- Salt and pepper to taste

Cooking Method:

1. Preheat oven to 300°F (150°C).
2. Heat olive oil in a large ovenproof pot over medium-high heat. Brown the lamb chunks on all sides, then remove and set aside.
3. In the same pot, sauté onion and garlic until softened.
4. Add the carrots, parsnips, broth, rosemary, thyme, salt, and pepper. Return the lamb to the pot.
5. Cover and bake in the oven for 1 ½–2 hours until the lamb is tender and the vegetables are cooked through.
6. Serve the lamb with the vegetables and broth.

Nutritional Facts (per serving): Calories: 450 | Protein: 35g | Carbs: 30g | Fat: 25g | Fiber: 8g

Substitution Variations:

- Use beef stew meat instead of lamb for a different flavor.
- Substitute root vegetables with other AIP-friendly vegetables like sweet potatoes or turnips.

Portion Control:

- A serving consists of about 4 oz of lamb and 1 ½ cups of root vegetables. Adjust the portions according to individual needs.

Pro Tips:

- For extra flavor, sear the lamb in batches to get a good caramelized crust.
- If you have time, marinate the lamb with rosemary and garlic for a few hours before cooking for more depth of flavor.

Coconut-Lime Fish Tacos (in Lettuce Wraps)

This recipe is a fresh and vibrant twist on tacos. It uses fish fillets wrapped in lettuce leaves, topped with coconut and lime, for a zesty, flavorful dish.

Estimated Meal Time:

- 25 minutes (prep and cook)

Ingredients:

- 4 white fish fillets (such as cod or tilapia)
- 1 tbsp olive oil
- 1 tsp ground cumin
- 1 tsp paprika
- Salt and pepper to taste
- 1 cup shredded coconut (unsweetened)
- 1 lime, juiced and zested
- 8 large lettuce leaves (such as romaine or butter lettuce)
- Fresh cilantro for garnish (optional)

Cooking Method:

1. Preheat a skillet over medium heat and add olive oil. Season the fish fillets with cumin, paprika, salt, and pepper.

2. Cook the fish for 3–4 minutes per side, until flaky and cooked through.

3. While the fish is cooking, toast the shredded coconut in a separate skillet over low heat for 2–3 minutes until golden brown.

4. Once the fish is done, flake it with a fork and place a portion in each lettuce leaf.

5. Top with toasted coconut, lime juice, lime zest, and cilantro. Serve immediately.

Nutritional Facts (per serving): Calories: 280 | Protein: 25g | Carbs: 12g | Fat: 18g | Fiber: 6g

Substitution Variations:

- Use shrimp or chicken instead of white fish.
- Add avocado slices for extra creaminess and healthy fats.

Portion Control:

- A serving includes 1 fish fillet (about 4 oz) and 2 lettuce wraps. Adjust according to hunger levels.

Pro Tips:

- Use a mild fish like cod or halibut for a more delicate flavor.
- For extra zest, add a squeeze of lime juice on top before serving.

Chicken and Spinach Stuffed Mushrooms

These hearty stuffed mushrooms are filled with a savory chicken and spinach mixture—perfect for an appetizer or a light dinner.

Estimated Meal Time:

- 30 minutes (prep and cook)

Ingredients:

- 8 large mushroom caps
- 1 lb ground chicken
- 1 tbsp olive oil
- 2 cups spinach, chopped
- 1 tsp garlic powder
- Salt and pepper to taste
- Fresh parsley for garnish (optional)

Cooking Method:

1. Preheat oven to 375°F (190°C).

2. Remove the stems from the mushrooms and set the caps aside.

3. In a skillet, heat the olive oil over medium heat. Cook the ground chicken until browned, about 8 minutes.

4. Add chopped spinach, garlic powder, salt, and pepper, and cook until the spinach is wilted.

5. Stuff the mushroom caps with the chicken and spinach mixture and place them on a baking sheet.

6. Bake for 15–20 minutes until the mushrooms are tender.

7. Garnish with fresh parsley and serve.

Nutritional Facts (per serving): Calories: 250 | Protein: 25g | Carbs: 10g | Fat: 15g | Fiber: 4g

Substitution Variations:

- Use ground turkey or beef instead of chicken for a different flavor.
- Add diced onions or bell peppers to the stuffing mixture for extra flavor.

Portion Control:

- One stuffed mushroom cap (about 3 oz of filling) is typically one serving. Adjust the portion to suit your appetite.

Pro Tips:

- If you want a cheesy flavor, add a sprinkle of nutritional yeast to the chicken mixture.
- These stuffed mushrooms can also be made in advance and reheated in the oven when ready to serve.

98

Pork Tenderloin with Apple and Sage

This savory and slightly sweet dish features tender pork, complemented by the flavors of fresh apples and sage for a heartwarming meal.

Estimated Meal Time:

- 45 minutes (prep and cook)

Ingredients:

- 1 lb pork tenderloin
- 2 tbsp olive oil
- 2 apples, cored and sliced
- 1 tbsp fresh sage, chopped
- 2 cloves garlic, minced
- 1 tbsp apple cider vinegar
- Salt and pepper to taste

Cooking Method:

1. Preheat oven to 375°F (190°C).

2. In a large ovenproof skillet, heat the olive oil over medium-high heat. Sear the pork tenderloin on all sides until browned.

3. Remove pork from the skillet and set aside. In the same skillet, add garlic, apples, and sage, and sauté for 2 minutes.

4. Place the pork back into the skillet and drizzle with apple cider vinegar.

5. After placing the skillet in the oven, roast the pork for 20 to 25 minutes, or until its internal temperature reaches 145°F (63°C).

6. Let the pork rest for 5 minutes before slicing and serving with the apple and sage mixture.

Nutritional Facts (per serving): Calories: 320 | Protein: 28g | Carbs: 20g | Fat: 18g | Fiber: 4g

Substitution Variations:

- Use chicken breast or turkey tenderloin as a substitute for pork.
- Add a handful of spinach or kale to the apples for more greenery.

Portion Control:

- One serving consists of about 4 oz of pork tenderloin and ½ cup of apple and sage mixture. Adjust the portion according to appetite.

Pro Tips:

- For added richness, drizzle a small amount of coconut cream over the pork before serving.
- This dish pairs well with roasted vegetables or mashed cauliflower.

AIP Beef Stir-Fry with Bok Choy

A simple and flavorful stir-fry featuring tender beef and nutrient-packed bok choy—perfect for a quick and satisfying dinner.

Estimated Meal Time:

- 20 minutes (prep and cook)

Ingredients:

- 1 lb flank steak, thinly sliced
- 2 tbsp olive oil
- 3 cups bok choy, chopped
- 1 bell pepper, sliced
- 2 cloves garlic, minced
- 1 tbsp ginger, grated
- 2 tbsp coconut aminos
- Salt and pepper to taste

Cooking Method:

1. Heat olive oil in a large skillet over medium-high heat. Add the beef and cook for 4–5 minutes until browned.
2. Remove the beef and set aside. In the same skillet, add garlic, ginger, bok choy, and bell pepper. Stir-fry for 3–4 minutes until tender.
3. Return the beef to the skillet and pour in the coconut aminos. Cook for another 2 minutes, allowing the flavors to combine.
4. Serve hot, garnished with extra ginger or sesame seeds if desired.

Nutritional Facts (per serving): Calories: 300 | Protein: 30g | Carbs: 15g | Fat: 18g | Fiber: 4g

Substitution Variations:

- Swap bok choy for kale or spinach.
- Use chicken or pork instead of beef for variety.

Portion Control:

- A typical serving consists of 4 oz of beef and 1 ½ cups of vegetables. Adjust based on your needs.

Pro Tips:

- For an extra boost of flavor, add a dash of garlic powder or chili flakes for a spicy kick.
- Serve with cauliflower rice for a complete meal.

Roasted Duck Breast with Caramelized Carrots

This elegant dish of roasted duck breast paired with sweet caramelized carrots is a delightful combination of savory and sweet flavors.

Estimated Meal Time:

- 1 hour (prep and cook)

Ingredients:

- 2 duck breasts
- 2 tbsp olive oil
- 4 large carrots, peeled and sliced
- 1 tbsp honey
- 1 tsp thyme
- Salt and pepper to taste

Cooking Method:

1. Preheat the oven to 375°F (190°C).
2. Score the duck breasts and season with salt and pepper. Heat olive oil in a skillet over medium-high heat, then sear the duck breasts skin-side down for 5–6 minutes.
3. Flip the duck breasts and transfer the skillet to the oven. Roast for 10–15 minutes for medium-rare.
4. Meanwhile, sauté the carrots in a separate pan with honey, thyme, salt, and pepper for 10–12 minutes, until caramelized.
5. Serve the duck breasts with the caramelized carrots on the side.

Nutritional Facts (per serving): Calories: 450 | Protein: 28g | Carbs: 25g | Fat: 30g | Fiber: 6g

Substitution Variations:

- Use chicken breast instead of duck for a leaner option.
- Add parsnips or sweet potatoes for additional root vegetables.

Portion Control:

- A serving consists of 1 duck breast (about 6 oz) and 1 cup of caramelized carrots. Adjust the portions according to preference.

Pro Tips:

- If you prefer crispy skin on your duck, increase the searing time before roasting.
- For a lighter option, substitute honey with a dash of maple syrup.

AIP Beef Meatballs with Zucchini Noodles

These savory beef meatballs are paired with fresh zucchini noodles for a healthy, grain-free, and satisfying meal.

Estimated Meal Time:

- 30 minutes (prep and cook)

Ingredients:

- 1 lb ground beef
- 1 egg (or egg substitute)
- 1 tbsp fresh parsley, chopped
- 1 tsp garlic powder
- 4 zucchinis, spiralized
- 1 tbsp olive oil
- Salt and pepper to taste

Cooking Method:

1. Preheat the oven to 375°F (190°C).
2. In a bowl, mix the ground beef, egg, parsley, garlic powder, salt, and pepper. Form into 12 meatballs and place them on a baking sheet.
3. Bake the meatballs for 20 minutes until cooked through.
4. While the meatballs are baking, sauté the zucchini noodles in olive oil for 2–3 minutes until tender.
5. Serve the meatballs over the zucchini noodles.

Nutritional Facts (per serving): Calories: 300 | Protein: 28g | Carbs: 10g | Fat: 20g | Fiber: 6g

Substitution Variations:

- Use ground turkey or chicken instead of beef for a lighter option.
- Add marinara sauce (AIP-friendly) to make it more flavorful.

Portion Control:

- A serving consists of 3 meatballs (about 4 oz of meat) and 1 ½ cups of zucchini noodles. Adjust based on hunger levels.

Pro Tips:

- For extra flavor, season the meatballs with onion powder or smoked paprika.
- Top the meatballs with a sprinkle of nutritional yeast for a cheesy taste without dairy.

Seared Cod with Lemon-Dill Roasted Potatoes

This light yet flavorful cod is paired with roasted potatoes, providing a balanced and satisfying meal.

Estimated Meal Time:

- 35 minutes (prep and cook)

Ingredients:

- 4 cod fillets (4 oz each)
- 2 tbsp olive oil
- 1 lemon, juiced and zested
- 2 tbsp fresh dill, chopped
- 4 medium potatoes, cubed
- Salt and pepper to taste

Cooking Method:

1. Preheat oven to 400°F (200°C).
2. Toss the cubed potatoes with 1 tbsp olive oil, salt, and pepper, then spread on a baking sheet. Roast for 20 minutes, turning halfway through.
3. While the potatoes are roasting, heat 1 tbsp olive oil in a skillet over medium heat. Season the cod fillets with salt, pepper, and lemon zest.
4. Sear the cod for 3–4 minutes per side until golden brown and cooked through.
5. Serve the cod with the roasted potatoes, drizzled with lemon juice and topped with fresh dill.

Nutritional Facts (per serving): Calories: 350 | Protein: 30g | Carbs: 30g | Fat: 16g | Fiber: 5g

Substitution Variations:

- Use any white fish like halibut or tilapia in place of cod.
- Add steamed broccoli or spinach for a vegetable side.

Portion Control:

- One serving consists of 1 cod fillet (4 oz) and 1 cup of roasted potatoes. Adjust based on individual needs.

Pro Tips:

- For a crispy texture, coat the cod fillets in a small amount of arrowroot flour before searing.
- To enhance the flavor, add garlic powder or paprika to the potatoes.

AIP Chicken Piccata with Sautéed Greens

A delightful AIP-friendly version of the classic piccata dish, this recipe pairs tender chicken with a zesty lemon sauce and sautéed greens.

Estimated Meal Time:

- 30 minutes (prep and cook)

Ingredients:

- 4 boneless, skinless chicken breasts (4 oz each)
- 2 tbsp olive oil
- ½ cup coconut flour (for dredging)
- 1 lemon, juiced
- 1 tbsp capers (optional)
- 3 cups mixed greens (spinach, kale, etc.)
- Salt and pepper to taste

Cooking Method:

1. Season the chicken breasts with salt and pepper. Dredge each piece in coconut flour, shaking off the excess.

2. In a skillet, heat the olive oil over medium heat. Cook the chicken for 4–5 minutes on each side, until browned and cooked through.

3. Remove the chicken and set aside. In the same skillet, add lemon juice, capers (if using), and a splash of water, scraping up any browned bits from the bottom of the pan.

4. Sauté the greens in the skillet for 2–3 minutes until wilted.

5. Serve the chicken over the sautéed greens with the lemon sauce poured on top.

Nutritional Facts (per serving): Calories: 340 | Protein: 30g | Carbs: 12g | Fat: 20g | Fiber: 6g

Substitution Variations:

- Use turkey breast or pork loin in place of chicken.
- Add roasted sweet potatoes or cauliflower rice to complete the meal.

Portion Control:

- A typical serving consists of 1 chicken breast (about 4 oz) and 1 ½ cups of sautéed greens. Adjust to your needs.

Pro Tips:

- If you like extra tang, add a teaspoon of apple cider vinegar to the lemon sauce.
- For an added crunch, serve with AIP-friendly crackers or a side salad.

Grilled Steak with Avocado Salsa

This flavorful and juicy grilled steak is paired with a refreshing avocado salsa that complements the rich, smoky meat.

Estimated Meal Time:

- 30 minutes (prep and cook)

Ingredients:

- 2 rib-eye or flank steaks (6 oz each)
- 1 tbsp olive oil
- Salt and pepper to taste
- 1 avocado, diced
- 1 small tomato, diced
- 1 small red onion, diced
- 2 tbsp fresh cilantro, chopped
- 1 lime, juiced

Cooking Method:

1. Preheat the grill to medium-high heat.
2. Rub the steaks with olive oil, then season with salt and pepper. Grill the steaks for 4–6 minutes per side, depending on desired doneness.
3. While the steak cooks, combine the avocado, tomato, onion, cilantro, and lime juice in a bowl. Season with salt and pepper to taste.
4. Let the steak rest for 5 minutes before slicing. Serve with the avocado salsa on top.

Nutritional Facts (per serving): Calories: 480 | Protein: 38g | Carbs: 15g | Fat: 32g | Fiber: 8g

Substitution Variations:

- Use chicken breast or pork chops instead of steak.
- Add diced cucumber or bell pepper to the salsa for extra crunch.

Portion Control:

- A serving consists of 1 steak (6 oz) and ½ cup of avocado salsa. Adjust portions based on personal preference.

Pro Tips:

- For extra flavor, add a sprinkle of chili powder or smoked paprika to the salsa.
- Pair with a side of grilled vegetables like zucchini or asparagus.

AIP Turkey and Butternut Squash Casserole

This comforting casserole combines lean turkey, creamy butternut squash, and aromatic herbs into a warm and filling dish.

Estimated Meal Time:

- 1 hour (prep and cook)

Ingredients:

- 1 lb ground turkey
- 1 medium butternut squash, peeled and cubed
- 1 onion, diced
- 2 cloves garlic, minced
- 1 tsp thyme
- 1 tsp sage
- 1 tbsp olive oil
- Salt and pepper to taste
- ½ cup coconut milk (full-fat)

Cooking Method:

1. Preheat oven to 375°F (190°C).

2. In a skillet, heat the olive oil over medium heat.
   Cook the garlic and onion for around five minutes, or until they are tende r.

3. Add the ground turkey and cook until browned, breaking it up with a spoon as it cooks. Season with salt, pepper, thyme, and sage.

4. Meanwhile, steam or boil the butternut squash cubes for 10–12 minutes, until tender.

5. In a baking dish, combine the turkey mixture with the butternut squash and coconut milk. Mix to blend.

6. Bake for 20–25 minutes, until the casserole is heated through and the top is golden brown.

Nutritional Facts (per serving): Calories: 350 | Protein: 28g | Carbs: 22g | Fat: 18g | Fiber: 5g

Substitution Variations:

- Use ground chicken or pork in place of turkey.
- Add spinach or kale for extra greens.

Portion Control:

- A typical serving consists of 1 cup of casserole. Adjust portion size based on individual needs.

Pro Tips:

- For a crispy topping, sprinkle AIP-friendly breadcrumbs or coconut flour on top before baking.
- This casserole pairs well with a simple side salad.

AIP Chicken and Cauliflower Rice Stir-Fry

This quick and easy stir-fry features tender chicken and cauliflower rice, making it a nutritious, low-carb meal that is both satisfying and flavorful.

Estimated Meal Time:

- 20 minutes (prep and cook)

Ingredients:

- 2 boneless, skinless chicken breasts, diced
- 2 cups cauliflower rice (fresh or frozen)
- 1 bell pepper, diced
- 1 zucchini, diced
- 1 tbsp olive oil
- 2 cloves garlic, minced
- 2 tbsp coconut aminos
- Salt and pepper to taste

Cooking Method:

1. Heat olive oil in a large skillet over medium heat. Add the chicken and cook for 6–8 minutes until browned and cooked through.
2. Cook the bell pepper, zucchini, and garlic in the skillet for a further three to four minutes, or until the vegetables are soft.
3. Stir in the cauliflower rice and coconut aminos, cooking for another 3–4 minutes until the cauliflower rice is heated through.
4. Season with salt and pepper to taste and serve immediately.

Nutritional Facts (per serving): Calories: 350 | Protein: 30g | Carbs: 18g | Fat: 20g | Fiber: 6g

Substitution Variations:

- Use chicken thighs or turkey breast instead of chicken breast.
- Add any favorite vegetables like spinach or mushrooms for variety.

Portion Control:

- A serving consists of 1 cup of stir-fry. Adjust the amount of chicken and cauliflower rice to suit your portion needs.

Pro Tips:

- For extra flavor, drizzle with a bit of lemon juice or sprinkle with AIP-friendly spices like paprika.
- This dish can be served with a side of steamed broccoli for added nutrition.

Lemon-Herb Grilled Shrimp with Asparagus

A fresh and light dish featuring succulent grilled shrimp with a bright lemon-herb flavor served alongside tender asparagus.

Estimated Meal Time:

- 20 minutes (prep and cook)

Ingredients:

- 1 lb large shrimp, peeled and deveined
- 1 bunch asparagus, trimmed
- 2 tbsp olive oil
- 1 lemon, juiced and zested
- 2 tbsp fresh parsley, chopped
- Salt and pepper to taste

Cooking Method:

1. Preheat grill to medium-high heat.

2. In a small bowl, combine the olive oil, lemon juice, lemon zest, parsley, salt, and pepper. Toss the shrimp in the marinade and let sit for 10 minutes.

3. Toss the asparagus with olive oil, salt, and pepper. Grill the shrimp for 2–3 minutes per side, and the asparagus for 4–5 minutes, turning occasionally, until tender and charred.

4. Serve the shrimp with the grilled asparagus and garnish with extra lemon zest.

Nutritional Facts (per serving): Calories: 280 | Protein: 35g | Carbs: 10g | Fat: 14g | Fiber: 5g

Substitution Variations:

- Use scallops or chicken in place of shrimp.
- You can also grill other vegetables like bell peppers or zucchini.

Portion Control:

- A serving consists of 4 oz of shrimp and 1 cup of grilled asparagus. Adjust portions based on appetite.

Pro Tips:

- Add a pinch of red pepper flakes to the marinade for a bit of heat.
- Serve with a side of cauliflower rice for a complete meal.

Baked Turkey with Root Veggies

This hearty and comforting meal features tender baked turkey paired with a variety of roasted root vegetables.

Estimated Meal Time:

- 1 hour 15 minutes (prep and cook)

Ingredients:

- 4 turkey thighs (or 2 turkey breasts)
- 2 tbsp olive oil
- 1 sweet potato, peeled and cubed
- 2 carrots, peeled and sliced
- 2 parsnips, peeled and sliced
- 1 onion, quartered
- 2 cloves garlic, minced
- 1 tsp rosemary
- Salt and pepper to taste

Cooking Method:

1. Preheat oven to 375°F (190°C).

2. Toss the root vegetables with olive oil, garlic, rosemary, salt, and pepper. Spread on a baking sheet.

3. Rub the turkey thighs with olive oil and season with salt and pepper. Place the turkey on the baking sheet with the vegetables.

4. Roast for 45 minutes to 1 hour, until the turkey reaches an internal temperature of 165°F (74°C) and the vegetables are tender.

5. Let the turkey rest for 5 minutes before serving.

Nutritional Facts (per serving): Calories: 400 | Protein: 35g | Carbs: 30g | Fat: 18g | Fiber: 7g

Substitution Variations:

- Use chicken thighs or a whole chicken for a different option.
- Add Brussels sprouts or cauliflower to the mix for more variety.

Portion Control:

- A serving consists of 1 turkey thigh (about 6 oz) and 1 cup of roasted root vegetables. Adjust based on hunger levels.

Pro Tips:

- For crispy skin on the turkey, increase the oven temperature to 400°F (200°C) for the last 10 minutes of cooking.
- Serve with a light salad to balance the meal.

AIP Chicken and Squash Frittata

A simple and satisfying frittata made with tender chicken and sweet squash, perfect for a nutritious breakfast or dinner.

Estimated Meal Time:

- 30 minutes (prep and cook)

Ingredients:

- 2 boneless, skinless chicken breasts, cooked and shredded
- 1 cup yellow squash, sliced
- 4 eggs (or egg replacements)
- ½ cup coconut milk
- 1 tbsp olive oil
- Salt and pepper to taste
- Fresh herbs for garnish (optional)

Cooking Method:

1. Preheat the oven to 375°F (190°C).
2. Heat olive oil in an ovenproof skillet over medium heat. Add the squash and cook for 3–4 minutes until softened.
3. Add the shredded chicken and cook for an additional 2 minutes.
4. In a bowl, whisk together the eggs and coconut milk, then pour over the chicken and squash mixture.
5. Put the pan in the oven and bake it for 15 to 20 minutes, or until the top o f the frittata is gently browned and firm.
6. Let it cool slightly before slicing and serving.

Nutritional Facts (per serving): Calories: 300 | Protein: 25g | Carbs: 10g | Fat: 18g | Fiber: 3g

Substitution Variations:

- Add spinach, zucchini, or mushrooms for more veggies.
- Swap chicken for turkey or pork.

Portion Control:

- A typical serving is 1 slice of frittata. Adjust based on preference.

Pro Tips:

- Serve with a side of mixed greens for extra vitamins and minerals.
- This frittata can be enjoyed cold, making it great for meal prep!

These recipes continue to provide a variety of delicious meals that adhere to the AIP diet while also offering portion control and flexibility for different dietary preferences. Enjoy!

<h1 style="text-align:center">Snack</h1>

Snack time can be delightful, nutritious, and completely AIP-friendly. These recipes combine creative flavors and simple ingredients to provide satisfying, energizing treats that support your health goals.

<h2 style="text-align:center">Sweet Potato Chips with Guacamole</h2>

A crunchy, creamy combination, this snack is packed with nutrients and flavor.

Estimated Meal Time:

- 20–25 minutes (prep and cook)

Ingredients:

For the chips:

- 1 large sweet potato, thinly sliced
- 1 tbsp olive oil
- A pinch of sea salt

For the guacamole:

- 1 ripe avocado
- 1 tbsp lime juice
- 1 tbsp chopped cilantro
- A pinch of sea salt

Cooking Method:

1. Preheat your oven to 375°F (190°C). Line a baking sheet with parchment paper.
2. Toss sweet potato slices with olive oil and sea salt. Arrange them in a single layer on the baking sheet.
3. Bake for 15–20 minutes, flipping halfway through, until golden and crispy.
4. Meanwhile, mash the avocado in a bowl and mix in lime juice, cilantro, and sea salt.
5. Serve the chips with guacamole on the side.

Nutritional Facts (per serving): Calories: 190 | Protein: 2g | Carbs: 28g | Fat: 10g | Fiber: 6g

Substitution Variations:

- Use plantain slices instead of sweet potato.
- Add garlic powder to the chips for extra flavor.

Portion Control:

- One large sweet potato makes about 2 servings.

Pro Tips:

- Soak sweet potato slices in cold water before baking for extra crispiness.
- Add a pinch of smoked paprika to the guacamole for a smoky twist.

Apple Slices with Coconut Butter

A simple, naturally sweet snack with creamy coconut butter and a warm touch of cinnamon.

Estimated Meal Time:

- 5 minutes

Ingredients:

- 1 medium apple, thinly sliced
- 2 tbsp coconut butter
- A pinch of cinnamon (optional)

Cooking Method:

1. Arrange apple slices on a plate.

2. Drizzle coconut butter over the slices.

3. Sprinkle with cinnamon if desired.

Nutritional Facts (per serving): Calories: 160 | Protein: 1g | Carbs: 22g | Fat: 9g | Fiber: 4g

Substitution Variations:

- Use pear slices instead of apple for variety.
- Swap coconut butter for sunflower seed butter.

Portion Control:

- One medium apple serves 1 person.

Pro Tips:

- Slightly warm the coconut butter for easier drizzling.
- For added texture, sprinkle shredded coconut over the apples.

AIP Plantain Chips with Salsa

Crispy plantain chips paired with fresh, tangy salsa—perfect for snacking or entertaining.

Estimated Meal Time:

- 25 minutes (prep and cook)

Ingredients:

For the chips:

- 2 green plantains, peeled and thinly sliced
- 1 tbsp olive oil
- A pinch of sea salt

For the salsa:

- 2 medium tomatoes, diced
- 1 small cucumber, diced
- 1 tbsp lime juice
- 1 tbsp chopped cilantro
- A pinch of sea salt

Cooking Method:

1. Preheat your oven to 375°F (190°C). Line a baking sheet with parchment paper.

2. Toss plantain slices with olive oil and sea salt. Spread them in a single layer on the sheet.

3. Bake for 15–20 minutes, flipping halfway, until crispy.

4. While chips bake, combine diced tomatoes, cucumber, lime juice, cilantro, and sea salt in a bowl.

5. Serve plantain chips with salsa for dipping.

Nutritional Facts (per serving): Calories: 180 | Protein: 2g | Carbs: 30g | Fat: 6g | Fiber: 5g

Substitution Variations:

- Replace plantains with zucchini for a lighter option.
- Add mango to the salsa for a sweet touch.

Portion Control:

- Two plantains yield about 3 servings.

Pro Tips:

- Use a mandoline slicer for uniform plantain slices.
- Cool the chips for a few minutes to enhance crispiness.

Tigernut Energy Bites

Delicious and portable, these energy bites are perfect for a quick snack or an on-the-go treat.

Estimated Meal Time:

- 10 minutes (prep only)

Ingredients:

- 1 cup tiger nut flour
- 2 tbsp coconut oil, melted
- 2 tbsp honey
- 1 tsp cinnamon

Cooking Method:

1. In a bowl, mix tiger nut flour, coconut oil, honey, and cinnamon until a dough forms.

2. Roll the dough into small balls.

3. Chill in the fridge for 15 minutes before serving.

Nutritional Facts (per serving): Calories: 90 | Protein: 1g | Carbs: 10g | Fat: 5g | Fiber: 3g

Substitution Variations:

- Add shredded coconut for extra texture.
- Replace honey with maple syrup.

Portion Control:

- One batch makes about 10 bites. A serving is 2–3 bites.

Pro Tips:

- Store bites in an airtight container in the fridge for up to a week.
- Add carob powder for a chocolate-like flavor.

Cucumber Slices with Avocado Dip

Refreshing cucumber slices with creamy avocado dip make a light and satisfying snack.

Estimated Meal Time:

- 10 minutes

Ingredients:

- 1 cucumber, sliced
- 1 avocado
- 1 tbsp lime juice
- A pinch of sea salt

Cooking Method:

1. Slice the cucumber into rounds and set aside.

2. In a bowl, mash the avocado with lime juice and sea salt until smooth.

3. Serve cucumber slices with avocado dip.

Nutritional Facts (per serving): Calories: 120 | Protein: 2g | Carbs: 8g | Fat: 9g | Fiber: 4g

Substitution Variations:

- Use zucchini slices instead of cucumber.
- Add fresh herbs like basil or dill to the avocado dip.

Portion Control:

- One cucumber and one avocado serve 2 people.

Pro Tips:

- For extra flavor, sprinkle cucumber slices with a pinch of sea salt.
- Serve the dip in a hollowed-out cucumber for a fun presentation.

Roasted Carrot Sticks with Coconut Yogurt Dip

Naturally sweet roasted carrots paired with a creamy coconut yogurt dip make a delicious and nutritious snack.

Estimated Meal Time:

- 25 minutes (prep and cook)

Ingredients:

For the carrots:

- 4 medium carrots, peeled and cut into sticks
- 1 tbsp olive oil
- A pinch of sea salt

For the dip:

- ½ cup coconut yogurt
- 1 tsp lemon juice
- 1 tsp fresh dill, chopped
- A pinch of sea salt

Cooking Method:

1. Preheat your oven to 400°F (200°C). Line a baking sheet with parchment paper.

2. Toss carrot sticks with olive oil and sea salt. Spread them out on the baking sheet.

3. Roast for 20 minutes, flipping halfway through, until tender and slightly caramelized.

4. Meanwhile, mix coconut yogurt, lemon juice, dill, and sea salt in a small bowl.

5. Serve the roasted carrot sticks with the coconut yogurt dip.

Nutritional Facts (per serving): Calories: 120 | Protein: 2g | Carbs: 13g | Fat: 7g | Fiber: 4g

Substitution Variations:

- Use parsnip sticks instead of carrots for a different flavor.
- Add garlic powder or smoked paprika to the carrots before roasting.

Portion Control:

- Four medium carrots make 2 servings.

Pro Tips:

- Roast carrots until slightly browned for a deeper flavor.
- Chill the coconut yogurt dip for 10 minutes to enhance its flavor.

Baked Kale Chips with Sea Salt

Crispy kale chips are a light and satisfying snack perfect for munching.

Estimated Meal Time:

- 15 minutes (prep and cook)

Ingredients:

- 1 bunch kale, washed and dried
- 1 tbsp olive oil
- A pinch of sea salt

Cooking Method:

1. Preheat your oven to 350°F (175°C). Line a baking sheet with parchment paper.

2. Remove the stems from the kale leaves and tear them into bite-sized pieces.

3. Toss kale with olive oil and sea salt, ensuring all pieces are evenly coated.

4. Spread kale on the baking sheet in a single layer.

5. Bake for 10–12 minutes, checking frequently to prevent burning.

Nutritional Facts (per serving): Calories: 80 | Protein: 2g | Carbs: 7g | Fat: 5g | Fiber: 3g

Substitution Variations:

- Sprinkle nutritional yeast on the kale before baking for a cheesy flavor.
- Add a pinch of chili powder for a spicy kick.

Portion Control:

- One bunch of kale makes about 2 servings.

Pro Tips:

- Ensure kale is completely dry before tossing with oil for maximum crispiness.
- Cool chips on the tray before serving to retain crunchiness.

AIP-Friendly Bone Broth Popsicles

A refreshing twist on bone broth, these savory popsicles are great for gut health.

Estimated Meal Time:

- 5 minutes (prep) + freezing time

Ingredients:

- 1 cup AIP-compliant bone broth
- 1 tbsp fresh parsley, chopped
- A pinch of sea salt

Cooking Method:

1. Mix bone broth with parsley and sea salt.

2. Pour the mixture into popsicle molds.

3. Freeze for at least 4 hours or until solid.

Nutritional Facts (per serving): Calories: 40 | Protein: 6g | Carbs: 0g | Fat: 2g | Fiber: 0g

Substitution Variations:

- Add a splash of coconut milk for a creamier texture.
- Use basil instead of parsley for a different flavor.

Portion Control:

- One cup of bone broth fills about 3 popsicle molds.

Pro Tips:

- Use silicone molds for easier removal.
- Let popsicles sit at room temperature for a minute before serving to make them easier to eat.

AIP Beef Jerky

Homemade beef jerky is a protein-packed, portable snack perfect for busy days.

Estimated Meal Time:

- 10 minutes (prep) + 4–6 hours drying time

Ingredients:

- 1 lb beef sirloin, thinly sliced
- 2 tbsp coconut aminos
- 1 tsp garlic powder
- 1 tsp onion powder
- 1 tsp sea salt

Cooking Method:

1. In a bowl, mix coconut aminos, garlic powder, onion powder, and sea salt.

2. Marinate the beef slices in the mixture for at least 30 minutes.

3. Preheat your dehydrator or oven to 160°F (70°C). Arrange beef slices in a single layer on the dehydrator trays or a baking sheet.

4. Dry for 4–6 hours, flipping halfway through, until fully dehydrated.

Nutritional Facts (per serving): Calories: 150 | Protein: 22g | Carbs: 2g | Fat: 6g | Fiber: 0g

Substitution Variations:

- Use turkey or chicken instead of beef.
- Add a pinch of smoked paprika for extra flavor.

Portion Control:

- One pound of beef makes about 4 servings.

Pro Tips:

- Store jerky in an airtight container for up to a week.
- Slice beef against the grain for tender jerky.

Coconut-Cinnamon Tigernut Granola Bars

These chewy granola bars are packed with AIP-friendly ingredients and natural sweetness.

Estimated Meal Time:

- 10 minutes (prep) + 20 minutes (baking)

Ingredients:

- 1 cup tiger nut flour
- ½ cup shredded coconut
- 2 tbsp coconut oil, melted
- 2 tbsp honey
- 1 tsp cinnamon

Cooking Method:

1. Preheat your oven to 350°F (175°C). Line a small baking dish with parchment paper.

2. Mix tiger nut flour, shredded coconut, coconut oil, honey, and cinnamon in a bowl.

3. Press the mixture firmly into the baking dish.

4. Bake for 20 minutes, or until golden brown.

5. Allow to cool fully before slicing into bars.

Nutritional Facts (per serving): Calories: 140 | Protein: 2g | Carbs: 16g | Fat: 7g | Fiber: 3g

Substitution Variations:

- Add dried blueberries for extra flavor.
- Replace honey with maple syrup.

Portion Control:

- One batch makes about 8 bars.

Pro Tips:

- Store bars in the fridge for longer shelf life.
- Toast the shredded coconut before mixing for a nuttier flavor.

Snacking on the Autoimmune Protocol (AIP) diet doesn't have to be boring or restrictive. These wholesome and flavorful snack options ensure you're nourished and satisfied between meals while staying compliant with the AIP guidelines. Whether you're craving something savory, sweet, or crunchy, these recipes provide a balance of taste and nutrition, supporting your health journey every step of the way.

Desserts

Indulging in dessert while following the Autoimmune Protocol (AIP) can still be a delightful experience. These dessert recipes are thoughtfully crafted to be both satisfying and compliant, using wholesome ingredients to create sweet treats that nourish your body and soul.

Coconut Mango Pudding

A creamy and tropical delight that pairs the richness of coconut milk with the natural sweetness of mango.

Estimated Meal Time:

- 10 minutes (prep and chill)

Ingredients:

- 1 cup ripe mango, diced
- ½ cup full-fat coconut milk
- 1 tbsp honey or maple syrup (optional)
- 1 tsp gelatin (optional for extra thickness)
- Fresh mint leaves for garnish

Cooking Method:

1. In a blender, combine the mango, coconut milk, and honey. Blend until smooth.
2. If using gelatin, dissolve it in 1 tbsp warm water and mix into the pudding.
3. Pour the mixture into small serving cups and chill for at least 2 hours.
4. Garnish with fresh mint leaves before serving.

Nutritional Facts (per serving): Calories: 180 | Protein: 2g | Carbs: 20g | Fat: 10g | Fiber: 3g

Substitution Variations:

- Replace mango with pineapple or papaya for a different tropical flavor.
- Add a pinch of turmeric for added anti-inflammatory benefits.

Portion Control:

- Serve in small ramekins or dessert cups to keep portions in check.

Pro Tips:

- For a creamier texture, refrigerate coconut milk overnight and use the thickened cream layer.
- Freeze leftovers in popsicle molds for a refreshing frozen treat.

Tigernut Flour Cookies

Soft and chewy cookies made with tiger nut flour, perfect for an AIP-compliant dessert.

Estimated Meal Time:

- 20 minutes (prep and bake)

Ingredients:

- 1 cup tiger nut flour
- ¼ cup coconut oil, melted
- 2 tbsp honey
- 1 tsp vanilla extract
- A pinch of sea salt

Cooking Method:

1. Preheat your oven to 350°F (175°C). Line a baking sheet with parchment paper.

2. In a bowl, mix tiger nut flour, melted coconut oil, honey, vanilla extract, and sea salt until a dough forms.

3. Scoop small portions onto the baking sheet and flatten slightly.

4. Bake for 10–12 minutes or until edges are golden.

5. Allow to cool before serving.

Nutritional Facts (per serving): Calories: 150 | Protein: 1g | Carbs: 10g | Fat: 12g | Fiber: 3g

Substitution Variations:

- Add cinnamon or ginger for extra spice.
- Use carob chips for a chocolate-like twist.

Portion Control:

- Limit to 2–3 small cookies per serving.

Pro Tips:

- Chill the dough for 10 minutes before baking to prevent spreading.
- Store in an airtight container to maintain freshness.

Baked Apples with Cinnamon and Honey

A warm, comforting dessert featuring baked apples with the fragrant sweetness of cinnamon and honey.

Estimated Meal Time:

- 25 minutes (prep and bake)

Ingredients:

- 2 medium apples, halved and cored
- 1 tbsp honey
- 1 tsp cinnamon
- 2 tbsp unsweetened shredded coconut

Cooking Method:

1. Preheat your oven to 375°F (190°C).

2. Place apple halves in a baking dish. Drizzle honey over each half and sprinkle with cinnamon and shredded coconut.

3. Bake for 20 minutes or until tender.

4. Serve warm, optionally topped with a dollop of coconut cream.

Nutritional Facts (per serving): Calories: 120 | Protein: 0g | Carbs: 30g | Fat: 2g | Fiber: 4g

Substitution Variations:

- Use pears instead of apples for a unique twist.
- Sprinkle chopped walnuts for added crunch.

Portion Control:

- Serve one apple half as a portion.

Pro Tips:

- Choose firmer apples like Granny Smith or Honeycrisp for best results.
- Experiment with additional spices like nutmeg or cardamom.

AIP Banana Ice Cream (Blended Frozen Bananas)

A simple, creamy, and naturally sweet dessert that requires just one main ingredient: bananas!

Estimated Meal Time:

- 5 minutes (prep) + freezing time

Ingredients:

- 2 ripe bananas, sliced and frozen
- 1 tsp vanilla extract (optional)
- A splash of coconut milk (optional, for creaminess)

Cooking Method:

1. Place the frozen banana slices in a blender or food processor.

2. Blend until the bananas become smooth and creamy, resembling soft-serve ice cream.

3. Add vanilla extract or a splash of coconut milk for extra flavor, if desired.

4. Serve immediately or freeze for 15–20 minutes for a firmer texture.

Nutritional Facts (per serving): Calories: 105 | Protein: 1g | Carbs: 27g | Fat: 0g | Fiber: 3g

Substitution Variations:

- Add a pinch of cinnamon or a dash of carob powder for a new flavor.
- Top with shredded coconut or fresh berries for added texture.

Portion Control:

- One medium banana serves one person.

Pro Tips:

- Use bananas that are very ripe before freezing for maximum sweetness.
- Store pre-sliced bananas in freezer bags for quick use.

Carob Coconut Truffles

These rich and indulgent truffles are a perfect AIP-friendly treat made with carob for a chocolate-like flavor.

Estimated Meal Time:

- 15 minutes (prep and chill)

Ingredients:

- ½ cup carob powder
- ¼ cup coconut oil, melted
- ¼ cup shredded coconut
- 2 tbsp honey
- 1 tsp vanilla extract

Cooking Method:

1. In a bowl, mix carob powder, melted coconut oil, honey, and vanilla extract until smooth.

2. Stir in shredded coconut.

3. Roll the mixture into small balls and place on a parchment-lined tray.

4. Chill in the refrigerator for at least 30 minutes before serving.

Nutritional Facts (per serving): Calories: 110 | Protein: 1g | Carbs: 8g | Fat: 9g | Fiber: 2g

Substitution Variations:

- Roll truffles in extra shredded coconut or carob powder for a decorative touch.
- Add a pinch of sea salt for a sweet-savory contrast.

Portion Control:

- Limit to 2 truffles per serving.

Pro Tips:

- Store in the fridge to maintain firmness.
- For a firmer texture, add a tablespoon of tiger nut flour to the mix.

Sweet Potato Brownies

Deliciously moist and naturally sweet, these brownies are a satisfying dessert option while staying AIP-compliant.

Estimated Meal Time:

- 30 minutes (prep and bake)

Ingredients:

- 1 cup mashed sweet potato
- ½ cup tiger nut flour
- ¼ cup carob powder
- ¼ cup coconut oil, melted
- 2 tbsp honey
- 1 tsp vanilla extract
- A pinch of sea salt

Cooking Method:

1. Preheat your oven to 350°F (175°C). Grease an 8x8-inch baking dish or line it with parchment paper.

2. In a bowl, mix mashed sweet potato, tiger nut flour, carob powder, coconut oil, honey, and vanilla extract until smooth.

3. Pour the batter into the prepared dish and spread evenly.

4. Bake for 20–25 minutes or until a toothpick inserted into the center comes out clean.

5. Let cool before slicing.

Nutritional Facts (per serving): Calories: 140 | Protein: 1g | Carbs: 18g | Fat: 7g | Fiber: 3g

Substitution Variations:

- Add chopped tiger nuts for a nutty crunch.
- Substitute mashed butternut squash for a similar consistency.

Portion Control:

- Cut into 9 small squares and serve one piece per portion.

Pro Tips:

- Use Japanese sweet potatoes for a slightly sweeter flavor.
- Store in an airtight container for up to 3 days.

AIP Strawberry Gelatin

A refreshing and naturally sweet dessert made with pureed strawberries and a healthy gelatin base—perfect for cooling off or as a light treat.

Estimated Meal Time:

- 10 minutes (prep) + setting time

Ingredients:

- 2 cups fresh or frozen strawberries
- 1 tbsp honey (optional)
- 1 ½ tbsp AIP-compliant gelatin
- 1 cup water

Cooking Method:

1. In a blender, blend the strawberries until smooth.

2. In a small saucepan, heat the water and honey (if using) over medium heat until it begins to simmer.

3. Sprinkle the gelatin into the simmering water and stir until dissolved.

4. Stir in the strawberry puree and mix well.

5. Pour the mixture into a mold or dish and refrigerate for 2–3 hours or until set.

Nutritional Facts (per serving): Calories: 60 | Protein: 2g | Carbs: 14g | Fat: 0g | Fiber: 2g

Substitution Variations:

- Use blueberries or raspberries for a different flavor.
- Add a few mint leaves or lemon zest for a refreshing twist.

Portion Control:

- This recipe yields about 4 servings.

Pro Tips:

- For extra smooth gelatin, strain the strawberry puree before using.
- Gelatin can be stored in an airtight container for up to 5 days in the fridge.

Apple Tigernut Crumble

This warm, comforting dessert combines tender baked apples with a crunchy, nutty crumble topping for a perfect fall-inspired treat.

Estimated Meal Time:

- 30 minutes (prep and bake)

Ingredients:

- 4 medium apples, peeled and sliced
- ½ cup tiger nut flour
- ¼ cup shredded coconut
- 2 tbsp coconut oil, melted
- 2 tbsp honey or maple syrup
- 1 tsp cinnamon
- A pinch of sea salt

Cooking Method:

1. Preheat your oven to 350°F (175°C).
2. Place the sliced apples in a baking dish, spreading them evenly.
3. In a bowl, combine tiger nut flour, shredded coconut, cinnamon, and sea salt. Stir in melted coconut oil and honey until the mixture resembles coarse crumbs.
4. Sprinkle the crumble topping over the apples and bake for 25–30 minutes, until the apples are tender and the topping is golden.
5. Serve warm, optionally with a dollop of coconut whipped cream.

Nutritional Facts (per serving): Calories: 160 | Protein: 2g | Carbs: 24g | Fat: 9g | Fiber: 6g

Substitution Variations:

- Use pears or peaches in place of apples for a different flavor.
- Add chopped walnuts or almonds for extra crunch.

Portion Control:

- This recipe makes 4–6 servings, depending on portion size.

Pro Tips:

- Use tart apples like Granny Smith for a nice balance of sweetness and acidity.
- You can prepare the topping in advance and store it in the fridge until ready to bake.

Coconut Milk Popsicles with Berries

These creamy, fruity popsicles are an easy way to enjoy a refreshing dessert while staying AIP-friendly. Coconut milk adds richness, while berries provide natural sweetness and antioxidants.

Estimated Meal Time:

- 10 minutes (prep) + freezing time

Ingredients:

- 1 can full-fat coconut milk
- 1 cup mixed berries (such as strawberries, blueberries, raspberries)
- 2 tbsp honey or maple syrup (optional)
- 1 tsp vanilla extract

Cooking Method:

1. In a blender, combine coconut milk, honey (if using), and vanilla extract. Blend until smooth.

2. Layer the berries in popsicle molds, then pour the coconut milk mixture over the top.

3. Insert sticks into the molds and freeze for at least 4 hours or until solid.

4. To release, run warm water over the outside of the mold for a few seconds.

Nutritional Facts (per serving): Calories: 120 | Protein: 1g | Carbs: 10g | Fat: 10g | Fiber: 2g

Substitution Variations:

- Add a handful of spinach or kale for a green version that's still refreshing.
- Use different fruit combinations, such as mango and pineapple, for tropical flavors.

Portion Control:

- Each popsicle is a single serving.

Pro Tips:

- Pour the coconut milk mixture in first, then gently press berries into the molds for an even distribution.
- Store popsicles in an airtight container in the freezer for up to two weeks.

Pumpkin Custard Cups

These creamy pumpkin custard cups offer all the warm, spiced flavors of fall in a silky, satisfying dessert that's AIP-friendly.

Estimated Meal Time:

- 10 minutes (prep) + bake time

Ingredients:

- 1 cup pumpkin puree (fresh or canned, without added sugar)
- 1 ½ cups coconut milk
- 2 tbsp honey or maple syrup
- 1 tsp ground cinnamon
- ½ tsp ground ginger
- ¼ tsp ground nutmeg
- 1 tsp vanilla extract

Cooking Method:

1. Preheat your oven to 350°F (175°C) and grease four small ramekins or custard cups.

2. Combine the pumpkin puree, coconut milk, honey, nutmeg, ginger, cinnamon, and vanilla essence in a bowl and whisk until smooth.

3. Pour the custard mixture evenly into the ramekins.

4. Bake for 25–30 minutes, or until the custard is set and a knife inserted comes out clean.

5. Before serving, allow it cool somewhat.

Nutritional Facts (per serving): Calories: 180 | Protein: 2g | Carbs: 22g | Fat: 10g | Fiber: 3g

Substitution Variations:

- For extra flavor, add a pinch of ground cloves or cardamom.
- Top with a sprinkle of shredded coconut or a drizzle of maple syrup.

Portion Control:

- Each ramekin is one serving.

Pro Tips:

- Store leftovers in the fridge for up to 3 days.
- To make ahead, prepare and bake the custards, then refrigerate to enjoy chilled.

These AIP desserts are not only delicious but also allow you to indulge in sweet treats while maintaining a commitment to healing and nourishment. Whether you're craving something creamy, fruity, or baked, these recipes provide the perfect balance of flavor and nutrition. Enjoy these treats as part of your autoimmune protocol journey, and feel confident knowing that each dessert is crafted with whole, nutrient-dense ingredients to support your wellness goals.

Chapter 7

Personalized AIP for Long-Term Success

Adopting the Autoimmune Protocol (AIP) can be a transformative journey, but it's essential to make the diet work for you for long-term success. This chapter will help guide you through fine-tuning your approach to AIP to ensure it remains sustainable, exciting, and tailored to your unique needs.

Listening to Your Body

One of the most powerful tools in your AIP journey is the ability to listen to your body. Everyone's experience with food sensitivities, inflammation, and healing is different. While AIP provides a solid framework, it's important to be mindful of how your body responds to the foods you eat.

Adjusting the diet based on personal needs:

- **Pay attention to your energy levels**: If you're feeling fatigued, it could be an indication that you need to tweak your diet, whether by adding more variety or reintroducing specific nutrients.

- **Notice any symptoms**: Keep track of any physical or mental changes, such as improved digestion or clearer skin, but also be mindful of flare-ups or discomfort.

- **Trust your intuition**: As you become more in tune with your body, you'll begin to identify which foods make you feel best and which ones might need to be avoided or reintroduced more slowly.

Remember, AIP is not meant to be a one-size-fits-all solution; it's a flexible tool to help you feel your best.

Fine-Tuning Reintroductions

After following the elimination phase of AIP, you may be ready to start reintroducing foods to see how your body reacts. This is a crucial step in personalizing your AIP journey. Reintroducing foods should be done slowly and methodically to ensure you can pinpoint any triggers.

When and how to retry foods:

- **Timing is key**: Wait for a period of time after eliminating a food before reintroducing it. Typically, you'll want to wait at least 3-5 days between each reintroduction to properly assess any changes in your body.

- **Reintroduce one food at a time**: This allows you to monitor your response to a single food without the confusion of multiple variables.

Start with small portions and gradually increase the amount if no negative reactions occur.

- **Track your reactions**: Keep a food journal to record how you feel after each reintroduction. Note any symptoms such as bloating, headaches, fatigue, or digestive upset. If you experience a negative reaction, it's best to remove that food again and try it later after your body has healed further.

The reintroduction phase may take time, and that's okay. It's a process of discovering what works best for your body.

Incorporating Variety

While AIP is an elimination diet, that doesn't mean your meals have to be bland or repetitive. One of the keys to long-term success is keeping your meals exciting and varied. This not only helps keep you motivated, but it also ensures you're getting a wide array of nutrients that support your healing journey.

Keeping meals exciting with new flavors and recipes:

- **Explore different herbs and spices**: The AIP diet encourages the use of healing herbs and spices like turmeric, ginger, and cinnamon, which add flavor and anti-inflammatory benefits to your meals.

- **Try new AIP-friendly ingredients**: Experiment with nutrient-dense foods like plantains, sweet potatoes, and a variety of leafy greens. You can also incorporate different cooking methods such as roasting, grilling, or slow-cooking to keep things interesting.

- **Make meal prep fun**: Preparing your meals in advance not only saves time but also gives you the opportunity to try new recipes and combinations of foods. Consider joining AIP cooking groups or exploring AIP blogs and cookbooks for fresh inspiration.

- **Get creative with AIP-friendly snacks**: Snacks are often the easiest meal to get stuck in a rut with, but there are plenty of delicious options to choose from, like roasted vegetables, fruit, or AIP-approved nut butters.

By keeping variety at the forefront of your meals, you'll stay engaged and energized throughout your AIP journey, preventing boredom and ensuring you enjoy the foods you're eating.

Incorporating these strategies into your AIP lifestyle will help you achieve long-term success. The key is to stay flexible, keep experimenting with different foods, and most importantly, listen to your body's needs. The Autoimmune Protocol is a tool to help you heal and thrive, but it's your unique journey that will ultimately guide you toward optimal health.

Chapter 8
The Science Behind AIP

The Autoimmune Protocol (AIP) is more than just a set of dietary guidelines—it's a science-backed approach to managing autoimmune conditions. In this chapter, we'll explore the research supporting AIP, its integration with functional medicine, and how it addresses the gut-immune connection, all of which contribute to its effectiveness in promoting healing and reducing inflammation.

Evidence-Based Research

There is growing scientific evidence supporting the effectiveness of AIP in managing autoimmune conditions and promoting overall health. Numerous studies have highlighted the relationship between diet and autoimmune diseases, showing that eliminating inflammatory foods can reduce symptoms and support the body's healing process.

Studies supporting the effectiveness of AIP:

- **Improved symptoms in autoimmune diseases**: Research has shown that people with autoimmune conditions like rheumatoid arthritis, lupus, and Crohn's disease often experience significant symptom relief when following an anti-inflammatory diet like AIP. Studies have demonstrated reduced pain, swelling, and fatigue, leading to improved quality of life.

- **Reduction in systemic inflammation**: Chronic inflammation plays a key role in the development and progression of autoimmune diseases. AIP focuses on eliminating foods that trigger inflammation and adding nutrient-dense, anti-inflammatory foods, which has been shown to reduce markers of inflammation in the body.

- **Gut health and autoimmune disease**: Studies have also pointed to the link between gut health and autoimmune conditions. AIP's emphasis on healing the gut lining and restoring a balanced microbiome has been supported by research suggesting that gut dysfunction is a common factor in many autoimmune diseases.

Though more research is needed to fully understand the mechanisms behind AIP, the existing studies offer strong evidence that dietary changes can have a significant impact on autoimmune health.

The Role of Functional Medicine

Functional medicine is a patient-centered approach to healthcare that focuses on identifying and addressing the root causes of disease rather than just treating symptoms. AIP aligns closely with functional medicine principles, as it emphasizes the importance of diet, lifestyle changes, and individualized care in managing chronic conditions.

How AIP integrates with other treatment approaches:

- **Holistic care**: Functional medicine practitioners often take a comprehensive approach, considering not just diet but also other factors like stress, sleep, and environmental toxins. AIP works synergistically with these other treatment modalities by addressing dietary triggers of inflammation while also supporting the body's natural healing processes.

- **Personalized treatment**: Just as functional medicine is tailored to the individual, AIP allows for customization based on personal responses to foods. This individualized approach is key to addressing the specific needs of people with autoimmune diseases, as each person may react differently to certain foods.

- **Focus on healing the root causes**: A functional medicine approach encourages healing the root causes of disease, such as gut dysfunction or chronic inflammation. AIP specifically targets these areas by removing foods that can irritate the gut and cause inflammation, creating an environment where healing can take place.

By integrating AIP with functional medicine, individuals can take a multi-faceted approach to managing autoimmune conditions, targeting the underlying causes rather than just masking symptoms.

Understanding the Gut-Immune Connection

The gut plays a crucial role in immune system function, and its health is directly linked to autoimmune disease development and progression. One of the central mechanisms behind many autoimmune conditions is **leaky gut syndrome**.

Explanation of leaky gut syndrome and its link to autoimmune diseases:

- **Leaky gut syndrome** occurs when the lining of the intestines becomes damaged, causing small gaps to form between the cells that line the gut. This allows undigested food particles, toxins, and other harmful substances to leak into the bloodstream, triggering an immune response.

- **The immune system's reaction**: When the immune system detects these foreign particles in the bloodstream, it launches an immune response, leading to inflammation. In individuals with autoimmune diseases, the immune system may mistakenly attack healthy cells in the body as it tries to defend against perceived invaders.

- **How AIP helps**: The Autoimmune Protocol is designed to promote gut healing by eliminating foods that can irritate the gut lining and cause inflammation. By following AIP, many individuals can repair the gut barrier, reduce systemic inflammation, and strengthen the immune system, helping to prevent the development or progression of autoimmune conditions.

Research has shown that addressing gut health is one of the most effective ways to manage autoimmune diseases. AIP's focus on nutrient-dense, gut-healing foods, combined with its elimination of foods that damage the gut, helps restore the balance of the gut microbiome and reduce the likelihood of autoimmune flare-ups.

The science behind AIP is grounded in research that supports its effectiveness in addressing autoimmune conditions through diet and lifestyle changes. By focusing on the gut-immune connection, functional medicine principles, and evidence-based practices, AIP provides a comprehensive approach to managing autoimmune diseases and promoting long-term health and wellness.

Chapter 9

AIP Meal Plans and Resources

Transitioning to the Autoimmune Protocol (AIP) can feel overwhelming at first, but having a clear plan and the right resources can make it much easier. In this chapter, we'll provide you with a practical 4-week meal plan, share some helpful resources for deepening your AIP knowledge, and guide you on how to work with healthcare professionals who understand the protocol. These tools will support your journey toward better health and healing.

4-Week Meal Plan

A meal plan is a great way to stay organized and ensure you're getting the proper nutrients while following the AIP. This 4-week meal plan includes delicious, easy-to-make recipes that will help you stick to your AIP goals. Each week is carefully balanced to provide variety and ensure you're getting a wide range of vitamins, minerals, and antioxidants. Along with the meal plan, you'll also find a comprehensive grocery list to make shopping simple and stress-free.

4-Week AIP Meal Plan

Week 1 Meal Plan

Day 1:

- **Breakfast:** Sweet Potato Hash with Avocado

- **Lunch:** Chicken Salad with Olive Oil Dressing

- **Dinner:** Herb-Crusted Chicken with Roasted Brussels Sprouts

Day 2:

- **Breakfast:** Chia Pudding with Berries

- **Lunch:** AIP Turkey Lettuce Wraps

- **Dinner:** Grilled Salmon with Garlic Mashed Cauliflower

Day 3:

- **Breakfast:** AIP Smoothie with Mango and Spinach

- **Lunch:** Tuna Salad with Avocado and Cucumber

- **Dinner:** AIP Beef and Sweet Potato Stew

Day 4:

- **Breakfast:** Coconut Yogurt Parfait with Berries

- **Lunch:** Zucchini Noodles with Shrimp and Avocado

- **Dinner:** Baked Chicken Thighs with Roasted Vegetables

Day 5:

- **Breakfast:** Banana Pancakes (AIP-friendly)

- **Lunch:** AIP Chicken Soup

- **Dinner:** AIP Braised Lamb with Root Vegetables

Day 6:

- **Breakfast:** AIP-friendly Smoothie Bowl with Mango and Coconut

- **Lunch:** Coconut-Lime Fish Tacos (in lettuce wraps)

- **Dinner:** Chicken and Spinach Stuffed Mushrooms

Day 7:

- **Breakfast:** Avocado Toast on AIP Bread

- **Lunch:** Pork Tenderloin with Apple and Sage

- **Dinner:** AIP Beef Stir-Fry with Bok Choy

Week 1 Grocery List

Produce:

- Sweet potatoes (3 large)

- Brussels sprouts (1 lb)

- Carrots (4 large)

- Apples (6)

- Avocados (4)

- Mango (2)

- Spinach (1 large bunch or bag)

- Cauliflower (2 heads)

- Zucchini (2)

- Fresh ginger (1 piece)

- Lemons (2)

- Garlic (1 bulb)

- Fresh herbs (parsley, rosemary, thyme)

Proteins:

- Chicken breasts (4)
- Salmon fillets (2)
- Ground beef (1 lb)
- Eggs (1 dozen)
- Canned tuna (2 cans, in water or olive oil)

Pantry:

- Olive oil (for cooking)
- Coconut oil (for cooking)
- Coconut milk (1 can)
- Coconut flour (1 bag)
- Chia seeds (1 bag)
- Tigernut flour (1 bag)
- Apple cider vinegar (1 bottle)
- Sea salt
- Black pepper
- Ground cinnamon
- Maple syrup (optional)
- Bone broth (1 carton)

Frozen:

- Frozen blueberries (1 bag)
- Frozen spinach (1 bag)

Other:

- Tigernut butter (1 jar)
- AIP-approved almond butter (1 jar)

Week 2 Meal Plan

Day 1:

- **Breakfast:** Sweet Potato Hash with Avocado

- **Lunch:** AIP Tuna Salad with Avocado
- **Dinner:** Grilled Chicken with Roasted Vegetables

Day 2:

- **Breakfast:** Chia Pudding with Berries
- **Lunch:** Chicken and Spinach Salad
- **Dinner:** Coconut-Lime Fish Tacos (in lettuce wraps)

Day 3:

- **Breakfast:** AIP Smoothie with Mango and Spinach
- **Lunch:** Zucchini Noodles with Shrimp and Avocado
- **Dinner:** AIP Beef Stir-Fry with Bok Choy

Day 4:

- **Breakfast:** Coconut Yogurt Parfait with Berries
- **Lunch:** AIP Chicken Soup
- **Dinner:** Baked Chicken Thighs with Roasted Vegetables

Day 5:

- **Breakfast:** Banana Pancakes (AIP-friendly)
- **Lunch:** AIP Turkey Lettuce Wraps
- **Dinner:** AIP Braised Lamb with Root Vegetables

Day 6:

- **Breakfast:** Smoothie Bowl with Mango and Coconut
- **Lunch:** Pork Tenderloin with Apple and Sage
- **Dinner:** Herb-Crusted Chicken with Roasted Brussels Sprouts

Day 7:

- **Breakfast:** Avocado Toast on AIP Bread
- **Lunch:** Chicken Salad with Olive Oil Dressing
- **Dinner:** AIP Beef and Sweet Potato Stew

Week 2 Grocery List

Produce:

- Sweet potatoes (3 large)

- Brussels sprouts (1 lb)

- Carrots (4 large)

- Apples (6)

- Avocados (4)

- Mango (2)

- Kale (1 bunch)

- Cauliflower (2 heads)

- Zucchini (2)

- Bok choy (1 bunch)

- Fresh parsley (1 bunch)

- Fresh basil (1 bunch)

- Fresh garlic (1 bulb)

Proteins:

- Chicken breasts (4)

- Salmon fillets (2)

- Ground beef (1 lb)

- Eggs (1 dozen)

- Canned tuna (2 cans, in water or olive oil)

Pantry:

- Olive oil (for cooking)

- Coconut oil (for cooking)

- Coconut milk (1 can)

- Coconut flour (1 bag)

- Chia seeds (1 bag)

- Tigernut flour (1 bag)

- Apple cider vinegar (1 bottle)

- Sea salt

- Black pepper
- Ground cinnamon
- Maple syrup (optional)
- Bone broth (1 carton)

Frozen:

- Frozen blueberries (1 bag)
- Frozen mango (1 bag)

Other:

- Tigernut butter (1 jar)
- AIP-approved almond butter (1 jar)

Week 3 Meal Plan

Day 1:

- **Breakfast:** Sweet Potato Hash with Avocado
- **Lunch:** AIP Tuna Salad with Avocado
- **Dinner:** Grilled Chicken with Roasted Vegetables

Day 2:

- **Breakfast:** Chia Pudding with Berries
- **Lunch:** Chicken and Spinach Salad
- **Dinner:** Coconut-Lime Fish Tacos (in lettuce wraps)

Day 3:

- **Breakfast:** AIP Smoothie with Mango and Spinach
- **Lunch:** Zucchini Noodles with Shrimp and Avocado
- **Dinner:** AIP Beef Stir-Fry with Bok Choy

Day 4:

- **Breakfast:** Coconut Yogurt Parfait with Berries
- **Lunch:** AIP Chicken Soup
- **Dinner:** Baked Chicken Thighs with Roasted Vegetables

Day 5:

- **Breakfast:** Banana Pancakes (AIP-friendly)
- **Lunch:** AIP Turkey Lettuce Wraps
- **Dinner:** AIP Braised Lamb with Root Vegetables

Day 6:

- **Breakfast:** Smoothie Bowl with Mango and Coconut
- **Lunch:** Pork Tenderloin with Apple and Sage
- **Dinner:** Herb-Crusted Chicken with Roasted Brussels Sprouts

Day 7:

- **Breakfast:** Avocado Toast on AIP Bread
- **Lunch:** Chicken Salad with Olive Oil Dressing
- **Dinner:** AIP Beef and Sweet Potato Stew

Week 3 Grocery List

Produce:

- Sweet potatoes (3 large)
- Brussels sprouts (1 lb)
- Carrots (4 large)
- Apples (6)
- Avocados (4)
- Mango (2)
- Kale (1 bunch)
- Cauliflower (2 heads)
- Zucchini (2)
- Bok choy (1 bunch)
- Fresh parsley (1 bunch)
- Fresh garlic (1 bulb)
- Fresh ginger (1 piece)

Proteins:

- Chicken breasts (4)

- Salmon fillets (2)

- Ground beef (1 lb)

- Eggs (1 dozen)

- Canned tuna (2 cans, in water or olive oil)

Pantry:

- Olive oil (for cooking)

- Coconut oil (for cooking)

- Coconut milk (1 can)

- Coconut flour (1 bag)

- Chia seeds (1 bag)

- Tigernut flour (1 bag)

- Apple cider vinegar (1 bottle)

- Sea salt

- Black pepper

- Ground cinnamon

- Maple syrup (optional)

- Bone broth (1 carton)

Frozen:

- Frozen blueberries (1 bag)

- Frozen spinach (1 bag)

Other:

- Tigernut butter (1 jar)

- AIP-approved almond butter (1 jar)

Week 4 Meal Plan

Day 1:

- **Breakfast:** Sweet Potato Hash with Avocado

- **Lunch:** AIP Tuna Salad with Avocado

- **Dinner:** Grilled Chicken with Roasted Vegetables

Day 2:

- **Breakfast:** Chia Pudding with Berries
- **Lunch:** Chicken and Spinach Salad
- **Dinner:** Coconut-Lime Fish Tacos (in lettuce wraps)

Day 3:

- **Breakfast:** AIP Smoothie with Mango and Spinach
- **Lunch:** Zucchini Noodles with Shrimp and Avocado
- **Dinner:** AIP Beef Stir-Fry with Bok Choy

Day 4:

- **Breakfast:** Coconut Yogurt Parfait with Berries
- **Lunch:** AIP Chicken Soup
- **Dinner:** Baked Chicken Thighs with Roasted Vegetables

Day 5:

- **Breakfast:** Banana Pancakes (AIP-friendly)
- **Lunch:** AIP Turkey Lettuce Wraps
- **Dinner:** AIP Braised Lamb with Root Vegetables

Day 6:

- **Breakfast:** Smoothie Bowl with Mango and Coconut
- **Lunch:** Pork Tenderloin with Apple and Sage
- **Dinner:** Herb-Crusted Chicken with Roasted Brussels Sprouts

Day 7:

- **Breakfast:** Avocado Toast on AIP Bread
- **Lunch:** Chicken Salad with Olive Oil Dressing
- **Dinner:** AIP Beef and Sweet Potato Stew

Week 4 Grocery List

(Refer to Week 3 Grocery List)

This 4-week meal plan gives you variety and flexibility while ensuring you're nourishing your body with AIP-approved meals. You can rotate meals if you prefer more variety or swap ingredients based on availability. The grocery lists for each week will help make shopping straightforward!

How to find AIP-knowledgeable doctors and nutritionists:

- **Look for functional medicine practitioners**: Functional medicine doctors are trained to approach healthcare from a holistic perspective, focusing on addressing the root causes of diseases like autoimmune disorders. Many functional medicine practitioners are familiar with AIP and can provide tailored guidance based on your specific health needs.

- **Search for registered dietitians specializing in AIP**: A registered dietitian (RD) with experience in AIP can help you plan balanced meals and ensure you're getting all the nutrients your body needs. They can also assist with reintroducing foods once you're ready and help monitor your progress.

- **Ask for referrals**: If you're unsure where to start, ask for recommendations from online AIP communities or local health groups. Many people who have successfully followed the protocol can refer you to professionals who understand AIP.

- **Consult with a naturopathic doctor (ND)**: Naturopaths often take a whole-body approach to health and are typically knowledgeable about dietary protocols like AIP. They can guide you through the process and offer support with supplements and other natural healing techniques.

Working with healthcare professionals who are familiar with AIP can provide you with personalized advice and ensure you're making progress while minimizing risks or deficiencies.

In conclusion, the right meal plan, resources, and professional support are essential to achieving long-term success with the Autoimmune Protocol. With this 4-week meal plan, valuable resources for deeper learning, and tips for finding knowledgeable professionals, you are well-equipped to manage your autoimmune condition and begin your healing journey with confidence.

Chapter 10
Maintaining Progress and Moving Forward

The Autoimmune Protocol (AIP) can be transformative, but its true power lies in the long-term commitment to your health and well-being. By focusing on balance, embracing progress, and setting clear health goals, you can continue your journey with confidence and clarity. In this chapter, we'll explore how to transition to a sustainable lifestyle, celebrate your victories, and keep moving toward your long-term health goals.

Transitioning to a Sustainable Lifestyle

The ultimate goal of following AIP is to create a lifestyle that you can maintain long term. While the elimination phase of AIP is often restrictive, the beauty of the protocol lies in how it can evolve with your needs as you progress. After completing the reintroduction phase, you may find that certain foods are manageable in moderation, and your diet can be adjusted to maintain both the health benefits and the joy of eating.

Balancing AIP with Everyday Life: As you move forward, it's important to find ways to balance AIP with the demands of everyday life. Social gatherings, dining out, and family meals can pose challenges, but with the right mindset and preparation, these occasions can be managed. Here are some tips for balancing AIP:

- **Plan ahead:** If you know you'll be attending a social event, take the time to prepare AIP-friendly dishes that you can bring. This ensures you'll have something to enjoy, even if the options at the event are limited.

- **Communicate your needs:** Don't hesitate to explain your dietary needs to friends and family. Most people will appreciate the effort and may even be willing to adjust dishes to accommodate your choices.

- **Gradual integration:** If you choose to incorporate non-AIP foods, do so slowly and mindfully. Listen to your body and monitor how it responds to the changes. This will help you make informed decisions about your diet while respecting your healing process.

Transitioning from strict adherence to the protocol into a more balanced lifestyle takes time, but it's a journey worth taking. It's all about finding what works for your body, your goals, and your lifestyle.

Embracing a Positive Mindset

The road to better health is rarely linear, and it's normal to encounter setbacks along the way. Whether it's a food reintroduction that doesn't go as planned or a busy week that throws off your routine, it's essential to stay positive and focus on your progress.

Celebrating Small Victories: AIP isn't just about eliminating foods from your diet—it's about fostering a deeper connection with your health. As you move forward, remember to celebrate the small victories. These could include:

- **Reduced inflammation** or fewer flare-ups

- **Improved energy levels**

- **Better digestion**

- **Enhanced mood**

- **Better sleep**

Each of these improvements, no matter how small, is a testament to the hard work you've put into caring for your body. Reflect on these moments and remind yourself of how far you've come. Celebrating the progress you've made not only boosts your confidence but also strengthens your commitment to your health journey.

Stay kind to yourself: Embrace the idea that setbacks are a normal part of any healing process. If you face a challenge, treat it as an opportunity to learn more about your body's unique needs. This positive outlook will help you continue moving forward with a sense of purpose and optimism.

Long-Term Health Goals

The final piece of the puzzle is setting long-term health goals. Whether you're using AIP to manage an autoimmune condition or simply to support overall well-being, it's important to envision the bigger picture and align your actions with your ultimate health aspirations.

Continuing the Journey Toward Better Health: While AIP can have immediate and transformative effects, true health requires ongoing commitment. Here are some ways to ensure that you maintain your progress and continue to build on your successes:

- **Revisit your health goals regularly:** Take time to reflect on your initial health goals and assess how you're progressing. Are you feeling more energetic? Are your symptoms improving? Keep track of your achievements, and adjust your goals as needed.

- **Prioritize self-care:** AIP is not just about food—long-term health is also about creating balance in other areas of your life. Consider incorporating practices such as regular exercise, stress management, and quality sleep into your routine. These factors will complement your diet and improve your overall well-being.

- **Stay connected:** Whether through a support group, online forums, or professional guidance, staying connected with others on a similar journey can help you stay motivated and informed. Sharing experiences and learning from others can be a valuable resource as you continue on your path.

Your health journey is not about perfection; it's about progress and finding what truly works for you. Every positive change, no matter how small, is a step forward. By committing to a sustainable AIP lifestyle, embracing a positive mindset, and setting long-term health goals, you're not just transforming your diet—you're transforming your life.

Moving Forward: Maintaining progress on AIP is about balancing dietary choices, being kind to yourself, and continually striving to improve your overall health. As you move forward, remember that each step—whether it's a success or a lesson learned—is an important part of your healing journey. With patience, persistence, and a positive mindset, you will continue to thrive and feel empowered in your health choices. Keep looking forward to the long-term benefits, knowing that each day is a step toward a healthier, happier you.

Conclusion

As you reach the end of this journey through the Autoimmune Protocol (AIP), it's important to reflect on the transformative potential this way of eating holds. AIP isn't just a diet; it's a lifestyle that encourages you to reconnect with your body, nourish it deeply, and take control of your health. It empowers you to address the root causes of inflammation and autoimmune symptoms, giving you the tools to heal and thrive.

Remember, healing is a process, and it unfolds over time. Each small, consistent step you take brings you closer to better health and wellness. Whether it's eliminating trigger foods, discovering new recipes, or learning how to listen to your body, every action contributes to the bigger picture of healing. It's not about perfection—it's about progress.

So, as you move forward on your path, take it one step at a time. Celebrate the small victories along the way and be patient with yourself when challenges arise. Healing is not a destination, but rather a journey—a journey that is unique to you and your body. Trust in the process, and know that with each new day, you're doing something powerful for your health and well-being.

You have the strength and resilience within you to continue this journey, and you don't have to do it alone. With the right tools, support, and mindset, empowered healing is within your reach. Keep going, and trust that you are making strides toward a healthier, more vibrant life.

Thank you for choosing this path. Your commitment to your health is the most important step you can take, and you are worthy of the transformation that lies ahead. Here's to a future full of healing, health, and empowerment.